Gift of Nature
WHOLE LEAF ALOE VERA
No. 1 Clinical Observations & Applications

HEALTH HAND BOOK SERIES
Written by Karen Masterson Koch, C.N.

Edited by Shelly Lewis, BA and Mary Carter, Ph.D., RN

Distributed by Total Health Science Press
Santee, California, 92072

Published by Westerfield Enterprises, Inc.
San Diego, California, USA

**Beyond Gluten Intolerance
GIS - Gluten Inflammatory Syndrome**

ISBN-13: 978-0-692-61650-3

Distributed by Total Health Science Press
Santee, California, 92072 USA

Library of Congress Catalog Card Number: 99-096727
ISBN: 0-942259-1-12-2

First Edition September 1999
Second Edition 2002
Third Edition 2005
Fourth Edition 2009
Fifth Edition 2013
Sixth Edition 2015
Seventh Edition 2020
Printed in the USA

Dedication

This book is dedicated to all of my patients who through their own tribulations of illness and their bravery to use health as medicine have reinforced the healing principles in my work and my life. Hope is the first step in healing oneself. There is no false hope. God Bless your efforts in getting well and staying well.

CONTENTS

Introduction... 7

From traditional writings to modern times, Aloe Vera can be used by children, adults, pets and the professional to support the immune system, wound healing and disease prevention.

Storehouse of Nutrients.. 8

Researcher Dr. Davis shows 15 important compound groups in Aloe Vera giving scientific basis for the over 1300 different worldwide research papers that have shown anti-inflammatory, antiviral and antibacterial support. Clinical observations from the results of taking Aloe Vera with; Cancer, Irritable Bowel, Asthma, Allergies, Chemical Poisoning and Prostate Cancer. Learn how to eat the actual Aloe Vera plant. Definitions of the different types of Aloe Vera products on the market.

Applications of Aloe Vera 35

Includes thirty-nine diseases of developing countries that Aloe Vera helps reverse, with support nutrients, diet and lifestyle guidelines.

Healthy Foods Diet Section 56

Diet #1 Daily Regimen - Foods For Health.
Diet #2 Regenerative Regimen-Candida, Low Blood Sugar, Herpes, Irritable Bowel Syndrome / Gluten Free, Allergies, Chronic Fatigue Syndrome.
Diet #3 Detoxification Regimen - Reverse Aging & Disease.

Food Diary 62

References... 63

A loe Vera is a high sulfur, green succulent plant, related to the Garlic family. Traditional herbal writings dating back to 1500 BC, have explained some of the mystery and applications of the Aloe Vera plant of years past. These writings describe Aloe Vera juice as a health tonic, to improve digestion while promoting rejuvenation and longevity. The Egyptians used Aloe Vera for centuries along with the Romans, Greeks, Algerians, Mexicans, Tunisians, Arabians, Indians and Chinese. Among the many medicinal uses, two very important applications of Aloe Vera were to fight infection and to use on burns. The Egyptian Queens Cleopatra and Nefertiti gave tribute to Aloe as one of their beauty secrets. Archeological evidence reveals the high regard ancient cultures placed on this plant. Images of the Aloe Vera plant, dating back to 4000 BC, have been found carved on Egyptian walls and coffins.

During modern times people are more aware of the topical applications of Aloe Vera rather than the therapeutic value of drinking the juice. The pulp and sap of the Aloe Vera plant have been applied to the scalp and skin through many different preparations. Improving skin conditions from acne, burns, bug bites, dandruff, wounds, psoriasis and even skin cancer have been reported.

New technical advancements in processing Aloe Vera in the last decade have provided higher quality products to be made for the world population. Recent scientific studies during 1987-1997 have isolated more specific applications for the *immune system, wound healing* and *disease prevention*. Drinking quality Aloe Vera juice and applying quality Aloe Vera products on the skin significantly helps the health of both animal and human population. With over 300 different species of Aloe Vera available the type, the process and also the amount of water in a formula will determine the medicinal results received from any given product.

The purpose of this handbook is to introduce all individuals; singles, families and the professional, to this ancient medicinal herb called Aloe Vera. By sharing my own clinical applications and scientific research, my hope is that you too, will begin to experience in your own life the *Gift of Nature,* Aloe Vera.

Aloe Vera, a storehouse of nutrients, contains 99% water. Over 200 active compounds available in the Aloe Vera plant are in 1% of the plant juice. Dr. Robert Davis, Phd., biologist-endocrinologist-researcher, states Aloe Vera contains 100 important compounds divided into 15 groups that work as a symphony to support health.

15 Important Compound Groups in Aloe Vera:

- Vitamins
- Minerals
- Enzymes
- Amino Acids (proteins)
- Fatty Acids & Uric Acids
- Saccharides (known as muco, mono & polysaccharides)
- Anthraquinones
- Sterolins & Sterols
- Lectin substances
- Lignins
- Gibberellins
- Saponins
- Salicylic Acid

According to Dr. Davis the biological activity or healing effects of Aloe Vera come from a synergistic modulation or "team effort" of all the compounds in the entire plant rather than from a single element. This explains why one herbal plant such as Aloe Vera can help so many different health conditions.

Functions of the Compound Groups in Aloe Vera:

Minerals, thirteen in Aloe, are responsible for growth and repair of cells in the body. Aloe Vera is especially high in the mineral sulfur. It is called nature's beauty mineral because it keeps the hair lustrous, the skin smooth and the complexion clear and youthful. Sulfur is paramount in collagen synthesis. Sulfur is a very important constituent of insulin, the hormone that regulates sugar metabolism. It also plays an important role in the energy metabolism of every human cell. Lastly sulfur stimulates the release of bile from the liver for fat digestion. When Aloe Vera is used both internally and externally, the high sulfur content may explain why it has so many beneficial effects for the skin, especially in the treatment of psoriasis and eczema. *Vitamins,* eight found in Aloe, are helpful to initiate important processes for daily metabolism of all systems of the body such as; digestive, nervous, lymphatic and the immune system. The *anthraquinone complex*, located only in the yellow sap of the Whole Leaf, contains aloin and aloe emodin. These two anthraquinones are responsible for bowel regularity. According to Dr. Davis, these constituents have other pharmacological properties such as anti-viral, anti-bacterial as well as anti-tumor activity. Several of the anthraquinones have also shown anti-inflammatory action.

Clinical observation of Anti-Tumor activity seen within just 2 weeks of drinking Aloe Vera:

Within the first few months of beginning the evaluation of a quality Aloe Vera juice in my practice, a young man named Andy with a confirmed lung tumor the size of a walnut, was referred to me by another female patient. A body builder by profession, he had harmed his immune system by taking steroids three years before our meeting. At that time he had developed a cancer growth in one of his testes and conceded to an orchiectomy. The doctors originally thought the surgery had removed all of the cancer growth. However, after this reoccurrence the doctors felt the lung tumor must have developed from cancer cells that traveled from the original site years before. Andy had not taken very good care of his health after the first go around with cancer. The doctors were convinced that chemotherapy should be started within two weeks along with a pre x-ray before starting the procedure.

I told Andy that I had been studying the effects of Aloe Vera on the immune system. The Whole Leaf Aloe Vera juice concentrate had actually revealed some tumor reduction in animal studies and from what I could see, it would not hurt him to drink it. He drank 3-4 ounces every day until his appointment. He also took 3000 mg.

ofEster Vitamin C and 50,000 i.u. of Vitamin A in fish oil form. He did not like eating vegetables yet I suggested that for these two weeks that he attempt to eat as many dark yellow, orange and green vegetables in conjunction with eating less meat and junk food. Since I had worked with Cancer for six years at the Livingston Clinic in San Diego, with hundreds of patients, I really did not expect much to happen in these upcoming two weeks. The call came from Andy, two weeks later. It was gone, he said. The tumor was gone! I honestly could not believe it. Yet when they did the x-ray to see just how fast it was growing, nothing was on the screen. And just like so many patients I have had over the years, of course, he wanted to know how long he would have to stay on this juice? I said to him, "Andy, first thank God, and secondly, if I were you, I would stay on the program for a year or longer, making certain to do a follow up with your doctors." Andy was the first of many cases to show the tumor reduction action from drinking Whole Leaf Aloe Vera Juice Concentrate.

Clinical observation of Whole Leaf Aloe Vera Juice Concentrate to prevent irritable bowel syndrome effects:

Patients are surprised when they come to me for a diet and they receive a program that begins reversing their disease. No one person has all the answers to disease yet a lack of health is always at the root of disease. Tim came to me to receive a diet for his severe case of Crohn's. Within a week of eating the foods on his new diet program for irritable bowel syndrome (IBS) and drinking Whole Leaf Aloe Vera juice concentrate, his symptoms all but vanished. He was back to work and feeling better than he had for years, in just a few weeks. The medical mind views stress, as the number one factor in developing irritable bowel. If stress was the cause of IBS, millions more would have problems with irritable bowel. Most doctors of today will acknowledge the wheat grain allergy with Crohn's. However, to understand all the factors and triggers associated with IBS; grains (gluten), dairy and sugar, the top three groups that cause the most symptoms and problems refer to page 57 - Diet 2 and the larger book, Beyond Gluten Intolerance – GIS, noted on inside cover page.   Many children have IBS along with adults. Even though the symptoms of indigestion and gas seem a bit minor at first, after years of the disease, the irritation that causes the upset actually promotes scarring in the intestines. This in turn may lead to a lack of absorption of nutrients from foods. It is a medical fact that one's health can deteriorate and even develop Cancer from a form of mal nutrition, that may develop from Crohn's or Irritable Bowel Syndrome (IBS). It is important to learn how to control and reverse this condition through diet and health programs. Advanced conditions of IBS can lead doctors to begin removing sections of the bowel that no longer function properly. They also prescribe cortisone derivative medicine that may have many undesirable side effects. Aloe Vera juice is a good preventative measure and may also be taken in conjunction with most medical programs. Reduce the daily amount of Aloe Vera ingested if loose stool or diarrhea. It is best to take with meals to support digestion and also stabilize blood sugar. See page 44-45.

20 amino acids are also present in Aloe Vera. Eight of the amino acids exhibit anti-inflammatory activity. Some show effectiveness with burns. There are 5 different *saccharides* in Aloe, known as monosaccarides and polysaccharides.

Definition: Mono means one, poly means many and saccharides refer to carbohydrate sugars. Polysaccharide is a molecular chain of many sugars. When the smallest size polysaccharides from Aloe Vera 50-100,000 Daltons, metabolizes in the body, it stimulates macrophages, which are cells that help the immune system function better. The reference to saccharide in the Aloe Vera research is actually referring to the polysaccharide. The first researchers in Aloe Vera termed these carbohydrate saccharides as *mucopolysaccharides*. This was due to the mucus like mucilage gel inside of the Aloe plant. Later this terminology was corrected, in that only animal forms of polysaccharides are properly called muco-polysaccharides.

Research on saccharides in Aloe Vera:

One of the 5 saccharides in Aloe Vera is called *mannose phosphate.* Dr. Davis demonstrated the effectiveness of this saccharide for wound healing, in the article published in the *Journal of the American Podiatric Medical Ass.*, 84 (1994): 77. The article called, "Wound Healing and Anti-Inflammatory Activity of a Related Growth Factor in Aloe Vera", told of very rapid healing with the use of Aloe Vera unlike other medical products on the market today.

Clinical observation of Aloe Vera healing wounds and leaving no scarring:

My patient Andrea, came to the clinic to learn how to stop eating sugar. She had just received a lumpectomy 6 months previously, for a breast tumor that was cancerous, yet her physician had not forced either chemotherapy or radiation on Andrea. She had read how eating a healthier diet could help build her immune system and needed some motivation and direction on how to improve her diet.

She was soon to have reconstruction surgery after her original tumor removal. Having had a fairly large tumor removed, the surgeon had to make an incision the full length of the breast from the chest wall to the nipple, approximately 6 inches long. I suggested to Andrea that she start applying a quality Aloe Vera juice to the incision, if it was not draining. She did so for about 8 weeks and drank 2 ounces of Whole Leaf Aloe Vera Juice Concentrate per day before meals. On her follow up visit she stated that drinking Aloe Vera and taking chromium picolinate, was helping her to stay away from eating so many sugary foods. The Aloe Vera seems to stimulate the pancreas to function more effectively for sugar metabolism. She also stated that her surgeon could not believe how fast she healed from the surgery. Andrea asked me if I would like to see her incision and I nodded yes. Viewing both breasts, I saw no scar on either one. I honestly could not see any incision what so ever. I was amazed once again with the healing qualities of Aloe Vera. She said her doctor had never seen anything like it either!

Immunity: Clinical observation of Colon cancer reversal with drinking Aloe Vera plus animal studies:

Another saccharide known as acetyl mannose, has received attention for its immune enhancing effect. Several scientific studies sponsored by Carrington Laboratories, first demonstrated the immune stimulation by this polysaccharide compound trademarked Acemannan, in vivo animal studies. The research was completed in 1990 at Texas A & M University and was supported by the U.S. Dept. of Agriculture and published in 1991, Vol. 3, June issue of Mol. Biother. The studies showed successful tumor reduction in research mice with implanted sarcoma cancer - through macrophage induced phagocytosis. All control mice not receiving the Aloe extract died in 20-46 days. 40% of the mice receiving the quality Aloe extract survived. This research proceeded the licensing of a pharmaceutical cancer drug, extracted from the Aloe Vera plant.

An interesting case was the aunt of our acupuncturist colleague who was on her third round of chemotherapy for colon cancer. Her doctor advised ending chemotherapy treatment after more cancer growth appeared. Dr. R. Warren OMD, asked about the special Aloe we had been using with our HIV patients for his aunt's health support? I told him it didn't look good for her yet since the doctors were giving up, it couldn't hurt.

Besides having her whole town praying for her, she began drinking 3 – 4 ounces daily of the Whole Leaf Aloe Vera Juice Concentrate, before meals. She went on 90% vegetarian diet, eating lots of vegetables, beans, low gluten grains and some fruits along with 3,000 mg of ester type Vitamin C, 400-600 mg of N-Acetyl Cysteine (NAC), Probiotics and 1-2 teaspoons of a daily greens supplement. Barely two months later I received a very sweet letter from Rick's Aunt telling me her doctors could not find any cancer. Just to extend one's life is success yet for this fortunate woman not a trace of cancer was left amazing us all.

Successful research on quality Aloe Vera exceeds 1300 papers including; immunity, auto-immunity, anti-inflammatory, asthma, diabetes, lowering cholesterol, antioxidant production, digestion and bowel health plus wounds, collagen and skin health.

Lectin substances found in Aloe Vera called *glycoproteins*, have been researched in Japan to reveal increased phagocytosis in support of lowering adult asthma symptoms and immune related actions. In 2018, Aloe polysaccharides demonstrated significant reduction in lung damage and other symptoms dose dependent caused by the Influenza - A Virus (N1H1) Infection in China's Shandong Agric. Univ. Tai'an, China. Thirteen different *enzymes* have also been identified in Aloe with one called Bradykinase that may play an important role to further reduce inflammation in allergies and asthma. Three *sterols* have also demonstrated a reduction in overall inflammation activity; B-sitosterol, Campesterol and Lupeol plus an aspirin like compound salicylic acid. *Lignins*, fibers found also in the Aloe Vera plant, may lower negative LDL cholesterol as well. Several research papers now confirm a quality Aloe Vera as the *"Director of the Butyric Acid Cycle"*, responsible for balancing immune function for bowel health and also supports a healthy autoimmune response, *Far More Than a Remarkable Folk Medicine: Aloe Vera and A. arborescens,* Yagi A, PhD, 2019. Quality Aloe Vera is truly the most important preventative step people around the world can take for daily body wellness.

Asthma has increased in the population and it is not only a nuisance in children and adults lives but a disease that kills. It is a condition that must be treated with diet and pharmaceuticals (as required) yet the side effects can be dangerous. Aloe Vera that has not been over-processed and containing the yellow sap seems to give the best support while decreasing junk foods and dry snacks which reduce trans-fats, sugars, cow milk and gluten that may worsen symptoms. Most patients received benefit from the health protocol (pg. 39) with the addition of a quality Aloe Vera and diet improvements. Vicky at age 10 loved to play soccer. Her Asthma was getting progressively worse to the point that family thought she might have to give up sports. Out of desperation she began drinking the Aloe Vera Whole Leaf juice concentrate (pg.39). On days when her breathing was more labored she took more. Vicky's episodes lessened greatly over the years with her use of Aloe Vera. She went on to graduate high school and played sports every year feeling healthy most of the time.

Clinical observations of drinking Aloe Vera to reduce allergies:

Allergies are irritants that enter into the body's environment and cause irritation in the blood stream. The medical community has no answers of how to rid one's body of allergic reactions. Medications can cover and help to control symptoms yet cannot stop the allergic reactions. Health regimens including a quality Aloe Vera juice can greatly support and stop allergic reactions entirely for many people, without any bad side effects. One important factor effecting allergies is the increase of a fungus in the body called Candida albicans. I have found that an overgrowth of Candida causes more mold allergy symptoms. The Candida can also block nutrient absorption from foods and inhibit the effects of medications to cause even more health problems. Many natural health practitioners view allergies as a stress disease. However, after using Aloe Vera with at least 100 different allergy sufferers, I believe allergies are primarily more of a digestion and absorption challenge. Drinking a quality, strong Aloe Vera juice daily will alleviate the symptoms of allergies greatly.

In my own family, Aloe Vera has helped allergies immensely! My daughter Dawn, a normal 13 year old girl, loved to shop yet she had many chemical allergies. Most common was the allergy to smoke, perfume and clothing chemicals. The allergies prevented her from shopping because the symptoms ranged from fatigue, dizziness, eye irritation and more. After just two weeks of drinking the Aloe Vera Whole Leaf juice concentrate, she noticed a big improvement. Eight years later she very seldom has a problem with clothing stores and she can now wear perfume when she chooses.

I have counseled a great many allergy patients to date. The improvements they have received vary from a reduction of sinus drainage, headaches, fuzzy thinking, digestive bloating and gas, skin rashes and fatigue, etc.. Many experience an abundance of energy from increased nutrient absorption. Foods that have caused previous digestive problems with irritable bowel become better tolerated. My husband Terry and younger daughter Loree, have also experienced amazing improvements from hay fever, animal dander allergies and miscellaneous sensitivities. Allergies are so wide spread in the world that it is no longer the question, who has allergies but who does not. Aloe Vera can be a blessing in everyone's family to enjoy the world we live in without being allergic to it!

Research on Diabetes; ulcers and wounds with (10) recent studies of Aloe Vera for internal support to pancreatic function (pg. 44, 54):

Gibberellin is a growth factor in Aloe Vera which may play a part in the wound healing process. Also, *Fatty Acids* are important in the body for growth and general health of all body tissues especially the skin. *Sterols* in particular are noted in many important pathways for anti-inflammatory action.

Many studies now conducted in the USA and abroad, confirm the astounding support of skin including diabetic ulcers, rashes and wounds applied topically from Aloe Vera. Research completed at the University of Cairo, appeared in 1973 in the publication *Dermatology*, Jan\Feb issue, Vol. 12 No.1, entitled "Use of Aloe in Treating Leg Ulcers and Dermatoses". A more recent study completed in the United States was chosen for presentation at the 12th Annual Wound Symposium in 1997 in Dallas, Texas. The 24 patients with 150 wounds, stages 1-IV, including a skin cancer, were treated with an Aloe Vera Wound Gel sponsored by Aloe Life International. The study entitled, "Clinical Evaluation of Full Thickness Wounds with Tunneling and Stage I-IV Wounds," showed 100% resolution of every wound, peer reviewed by the Springhouse Corporation's medical review board of doctors and nurses. (See page 17 & 55.)

Salicylic Acid is a natural aspirin like compound found in Aloe Vera. It works as an analgesic, which reduces pain and also exhibits anti-inflammatory support to damaged tissue. *Saponins* present in Aloe Vera are visible when a quality Aloe Vera juice is shaken and little bubbles appear. Saponins are molecularly referred to as *glycosides*. Glycosides exhibit an antiseptic quality in the body and provide a natural fortifier when applied to the hair, giving new life and body to the hair shaft. The saponins may have antibacterial action against staph.

Wound Healing with Aloe Vera - R. H. Davis, Ph. D.

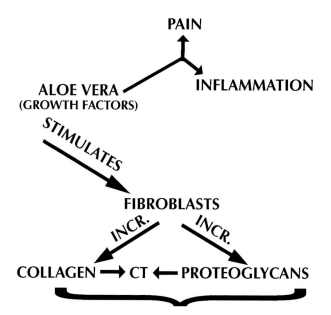

PAIN

ALOE VERA
(GROWTH FACTORS)

INFLAMMATION

STIMULATES

FIBROBLASTS

INCR.   *INCR.*

COLLAGEN → CT ← PROTEOGLYCANS

INCREASES WOUND TENSILE STRENGTH

Coccyx Case Study #20

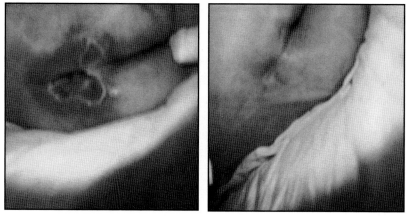

20 Days   141 Days

Aloe Life International 18 month wound study 1997

It is easy to see after learning more about the actives in Aloe Vera, why quality Aloe Vera has become the most popular choice for herbal treatment in modern America and around the world. In surveys of American health food stores, Aloe Vera sales were 1st place in 2009 and have stayed in the top 6th most popular - above hundreds of other herbs and super foods for topical and internal daily use. Safety studies support the use for children, pets and adults. The caution is to take Aloe Vera with meals and if diarrhea results reduce the daily amounts.

Global Research of Aloe Vera and Herbs:

Global research is on going with many herbal plants including Aloe Vera. Using portions of herbs in prescription medications is not new. In the 1950's close to 50% of all prescription medication were derived from herbal extracts. Two billion prescription drug medicines filled in the United States each year contain plant derivatives such as alkaloids, glycosides, steroids, etc. A good example of a drug sold in the United States derived from the herb Foxglove, by prescription only, is Digitalis. Digitalis, is used by people who have congestive heart disease. It contains several glycosides. The glycoside *digitoxin* is the one primarily responsible for foxglove's helpful action on the heart. Digitalis increases the force of heart contractions, which helps to empty the blood from the ventricle section of the heart. This gives the heart time to rest between contractions and to fill up again with blood from the veins. This in turn helps to reduce blood pressure in the veins, benefiting hypertensive heart disease. The improved circulation alleviates water retention and reduces edema in the limbs. The drug, derived from Grecian Foxglove Digitalis lanata has been used widely since the late 1940's. Foxglove should be used with caution and best to be supervised by a physician.

Countries participating in Aloe Vera research besides the United States include the United Kingdom, Russia, Egypt, China, South Korea, Japan and Germany. Dr. Lawrence Plaskett, a researcher and respected health educator, earned his Ph.D. in biochemistry at Cambridge University in England. After extensive research into the broad-spectrum remedy herb Aloe Vera, he reported in 1996 that over 200 peer reviewed scientific papers collected worldwide have been published from research on Aloe Vera during the past 20 years. The categories of research on Aloe Vera, showed support for the following.

Categories of 200 Worldwide Scientific Research Papers Published

- Anti-inflammatory Action
- Anti-bacterial Action
- Anti-viral Action

These pathways of action in the Aloe Vera plant translate into many applications for the consumer, including reduction of pain, scarring and excelerated healing of external and internal tissue for a multitude of conditions. These include; arthritis, allergies, asthma, hepatitis, ulcers, cardiovascular disease, diabetes, fighting infections, digestion, bowel disorders, dentistry, fungal infections, chronic fatigue, fibromyalgia and promising support for the immune and auto immune system. Dr. Plaskett's book, "The Health and Medical Use of Aloe Vera", 1996, Life Sciences Press, Tacoma, WA., elaborates on many of the studies that prove the value of using the natural remedy Aloe Vera. New research reveals Aloe Vera's **Transfer Factor** up to 300%.

Caution of Use with Aloe Vera:

Most individuals have no sensitivity to drinking Aloe Vera products or putting the plant gel on their skin. In fact for many people it improves their existing allergies 100%. See the allergy section. The occurrence of an actual allergy to Aloe Vera is rare, yet I have met three individuals in fourteen years of studying the plant, that developed a scratchy throat and a slight skin reaction with its use. It is wise, especially with young children and infants, to always do a skin test with any product, including Aloe Vera, to see if the ingredients agree with the individuals biology. If no rash or irritation occurs, after applying some of a product to the skin, then usually it will not cause any irritation when the juice is consumed.

However, each individual Aloe Vera company, that processes the plant, can use a variety of different stabilizers or preservatives to maintain the freshness of a product. The United States FDA (food and drug association), approves the food grade preservatives that are safe for the consumer including; sodium benzoate, potassium sorbate, citric acid, and ascorbic acid. It is my experience that these naturally produced additives have absolutely no harmful side effects. In fact one laboratory test showed table salt, sodium chloride, to have more harmful effects on cell health than these approved stabilizers. They are used only to prevent mold growth in the juice. Tests have shown that the body excretes both sodium benzoate and potassium sorbate from the body within 48 hours. Aloe Vera being a highly perishable vegetable juice must have some form of stabilization to prevent spoilage. It is not possible to put quality Aloe Vera juice in a bottle and keep it fresh without either 1.) high heat pasteurization or 2.) flash heat pasteurization (referred to as cold processed) combined with safe food grade preservatives. 3) Lastly irradiation.

Companies that state no heat and no preservatives on their labels, have yet to explain their ability to stabilize their aloe products and are suspect for processing ethics. The high perishability spoilage nature of Aloe Vera, is the primary reason the secrets of Aloe are now just unfolding to the mainstream consumer. Both quality and potency in Aloe Vera products have varied greatly over the past thirty years. Much of the traditional herbal testimonies have come from using the actual plant itself and not from using poorly processed Aloe Vera products.

Sulfites: If you are sensitive to sulfites or have many allergies currently, you will be interested to know that some companies do use sulfites in processing Aloe Vera. Sulfites keep the juice from turning darker in color. It is best to purchase Aloe Vera from healthfood stores that have more knowledge about the Aloe Vera companies processing methods. Consumers sensitive to sulfites will have a variety of symptoms ranging from headaches to disorientation, mood swings, fatigue and even gastrointestinal upset. Aloe Vera consumption alone does not give these types of symptoms. Quality Aloe Vera companies that are knowledgeable in health, would never use this very highly allergic substance in processing Aloe Vera. Products more golden in color will not generally contain sulfites.

Toxicity Study on Aloe Vera showed 100% safe:

This first controlled study to test any potential toxicity of drinking Aloe Vera on mammals was completed in 1997. Of the hundreds of scientific studies that have been completed on Aloe Vera, none have been for the sole purpose of checking the potential toxicity of drinking daily amounts of Aloe Vera over a long period of time. The 360, Fisher 344 type, laboratory mice, were the chosen mammals for this four year study. The control mice not receiving the daily Aloe Vera were fed exactly the same chemically balanced diet, as the mice given the daily dose of Aloe Vera. All of the scientific biological markers were monitored for the outcome. The results were very dynamic! The study resulted in 100% absence of toxicity. Not only did the Aloe Vera fed mice not experience any negative side effects, they also experienced much lower incidences of normal mice diseases. The scientists observed a much lower incidence of mice leukemia cancer. Kidney disease, commonly seen with mice was also remarkably lower with the Aloe Vera fed mice along with a significantly lower incidence of certain cardiovascular heart disease. "This was the first study ever performed using the long term feeding of aloe." says Dr. Byung Pal Yu, professor of physiology at the Health Science Center of the University of San Antonio, Texas. "As we reviewed all of the material data from the four year study, we found no toxicity and quite the contrary. The Aloe Vera fed mice lived approximately 25% longer than the mice not given the Aloe Vera!"

Scientific research results of mammals drinking Aloe Vera daily revealed:

- No toxicity in drinking Aloe Vera daily over long periods of time.
- Significantly lower incidence of kidney disease, leukemia cancer & heart disease.
- Increased life span of 15% in the animal group drinking Aloe Vera.

When Dr. Yu was asked in an interview at the I.A.S.C. world symposium on Aloe Vera, what active ingredient in the Aloe Vera plant was responsible for the life extension seen in this study, he laughed and said, "Aloe juice has many active ingredients. I have isolated only two myself, one being an antioxidant and another an anti-inflammatory agent. Someday with more research on Aloe Vera I hope to be able to tell you why this plant can extend life!"

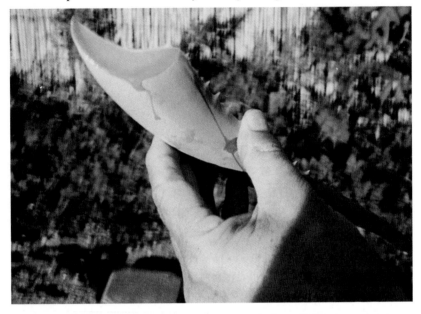

Can you eat the Aloe Vera plant without processing?

Yes, the Aloe Vera plant is edible yet some species are not as pleasant tasting as others. The Barbadensis Miller variety of Aloe Vera is pleasant tasting (inner gel only). If allergy has been ruled out, it is 100% safe to eat or use directly on the skin. In fact many people of Mexico and South America, have grown up eating the inner gel directly out of the plant. They also mix it, with juice or food, for a daily supplement to stay well. Mashing the inner gel and applying the sticky substance onto the skin, scalp and hair is common to restore health and promote hair growth. Only strong Whole Leaf Aloe Vera products can help hair growth in this manner and must be applied to the scalp daily. Drinking Aloe Vera juice supports hair growth as well. Sabila is the Spanish word for Aloe Vera. When I speak to people that know of Sabila, they grin from ear to ear. Sabila is respected like a family friend because of its wonderful regenerative and healing support.

How to prepare the Aloe Vera leaf for use:

- Make certain you have an Aloe Vera plant. The Barbadensis Miller variety has more pulp and not as much of the bitter property called anthraquinone as some of the species of Aloe Vera. It resembles a cactus with lance shaped leaves. The elongated leaves have sharp spikes along the scalloped edges. It is not a cactus however. The plant is in the lily family and blooms with yellow blossoms on a plumage out of the center of the clustered plant.

- Cut the entire outer leaf off at the base of the plant. Mature plants growing in the ground for 3 or more years will develop larger amounts of active ingredients including more of the yellow sap. The sap contains a very strong pungent odor very similar to strong body odor. Under developed plants grown inside have less of the yellow sap and smaller amounts of the therapeutic compounds. Healthy plants require sufficient sun, water, quality soil and wind to produce maximum therapeutic compounds.

- Wash the leaf well in water and split the leaf open, as one might fillet a fish. To avoid deterioration store any unused portion of the leaf in refrigeration.

- Carefully, scoop the inner gel out with a spoon avoiding too much of the yellow bitter sap located on the underside skin of the leaf. This has a very bitter, pungent taste and will cause diarrhea if consumed in large amounts.

- The inner gel can be eaten off the spoon or mixed in any beverage. The mashed inner gel can be applied topically as desired.

Note: The outer leaf of the Aloe Vera plant can be eaten by some hardy individuals yet the taste is very strong and may cause abdominal discomfort, cramping and diarrhea. I met a man from Mexico that said he ate a half an inch by two inch piece, of the whole leaf Aloe Vera daily and he recovered from his prostate cancer. No controlled studies have been conducted to replicate his testimony yet it made an impression of how medicinal Aloe Vera may be.

Folklore dictates that pregnant women might give birth prematurely by ingesting the outer leaf. The taste of the leaf is so repulsive that the chance of this occurring is very remote. All individuals need to use caution with ingesting the plant itself because of its laxative properties. The outer leaf or whole leaf constituents, are safely and easily consumed through processed quality Whole Leaf Aloe Vera products. The Aloe Vera companies remove varying amounts of the bitter laxative properties from the outer leaf through processing while maintaining most of the therapeutic compounds.

Important note: It has been written concerning pregnant women, children and seniors that they need to avoid the use of all Aloe Vera products. This is not a true statement. On the contrary, processed Aloe Vera juices including the whole leaf products are 100% *safe* for pregnant women, children, adults, seniors and pets. In fact children and seniors may benefit more than other age groups because of the greater need for immune and digestive support.

Major processing methods of Aloe Vera Juice

The two major processing methods of the Aloe Vera juice are:
• Fillet method
• Whole Leaf method

The oldest method is filleting which removes the outer leaf, rind and yellow sap, utilizing only the inner gel mucilage of the plant. New technology has enhanced the processing method of the Whole Leaf in recent years. This includes the entire leaf of the plant which contains 12% more total solids than the Fillet method. The solids in the whole leaf include 3-5 times more of the valuable polysaccharides that may play an important role in support for the immune system, anti-inflammatory support of the joints and glandular health. Since quality whole leaf Aloe Vera products contain much more of the active compounds in the solids, than the inner gel alone, the consumer receives much more benefit with the whole leaf products if they are processed properly.

Important factors in processing quality Aloe Vera products are:

• Harvested leaves must be processed within 3-6 hours of being cut from the plant or put in refrigeration. This reduces the natural oxidation of the leaves and will maintain an important laboratory marker called E-peak. This shows freshness and activity of the plant juice.

• Proper stabilization of processing through either High Heat Pasteurization or Flash Heat (Cold Processing) with the addition of an approved preservative system to prevent spoilage. This cold processing method uses flash heat which kills potential pathogens without destroying the life giving nutrients in the Aloe Vera such as enzymes, vitamins, and polysaccharides. Raw unstabilized Aloe Vera juice cannot be bottled for consumption.

All Aloe Vera products are not Aloe:

Aloe Vera juice is extremely therapeutic. Even a small amount of juice will give the consumer results. The stronger quality undiluted products, will give more dramatic health results. Some companies use more water than Aloe Vera in their end products and do not always list water in the ingredients. The Aloe Vera governing council is called the IASC, International Aloe Science Council. With the support of other health agencies, the IASC is helping to rid the market of dishonest marketing companies. However the IASC Certification is rather lax itself. To date they only require Aloe Vera products to contain 15% Aloe Vera for certification and do not require water to be listed in the ingredients.

Consumers Beware: When you see very low pricing of Aloe Vera products, testing results have shown that not much Aloe Vera is in them! Also I suggest that if you are not receiving the benefit from a chosen Aloe Vera product anticipated, use a higher quality product before assuming the herb just did not work. An example of this was a gentleman taking a low cost Aloe Vera product for his stomach ulcer. He felt better using the product regularly yet the ulcer did not resolve. A friend told him about a more therapeutic brand of Aloe Vera and his ulcer cleared up 100%.

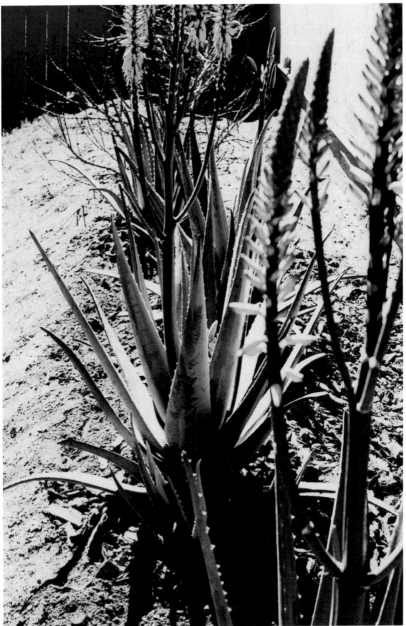

Barbadensis Miller Aloe Vera

Surprisingly, Aloe Vera processed with high heat does not loose all of the active ingredients. The heat does however break down the chemical bonds of the valuable polysaccharides and destroys vitamins and enzymes. Researchers say that only when these bonds are very small, intact at 80,000 to 400,000 Dalton size, will they stimulate the immune system. Quick processing from the field and the use of Cold Processing (flash heat) method, will maintain more of the enzymes and the polysaccharide bonds to support the immune system pathway of action. One new testing method called Active Aloe guarantees the polysaccharide activity in a product.

How does Aloe Vera Taste?

The Aloe Vera plant is a high mineral containing vegetable herb. It contains high amounts of sulfur, potassium (salty taste), Calcium and Magnesium along with an abundance of trace minerals. When undiluted, the consumer will taste these minerals in the juice. The inner gel does not have a strong taste because of the lower levels of solids. The strongest of the Aloe Vera products, Whole Leaf juice concentrate, taste similar to tomato juice, without the thickness or red color. Also the Aloe Vera plant has a natural chemistry pH, of acidic, similar to the pH of skin, ranging from 3.5-5.7. This adds to the slightly bitter taste along with the pungent yellow sap of the whole leaf juice products. These two properties are primarily responsible for the great improvement in digestion experienced by most consumers. Products diluted with water loose the natural herbal bitter quality because water is alkaline not acidic. If a product taste like water, regardless of the ingredients listed, it generally has more water than Aloe in the product.

Aloe Vera tablets or capsules should also have a similar taste of minerals not a sweet taste. If any Aloe Vera product tastes sweet, it is from the refined sugar added during the drying process called maltose dextrin. Some powdered Aloe Vera can contain up to 50% sugar. Manufacturers may also add fillers to extend the Aloe Vera used in capsules or tablets. If a product is pure and made from the whole leaf, a bitter almost pungent taste will always be present, not sweet.

When is the best time to drink Aloe Vera juice?

The consumer can drink the Aloe Vera juice straight out of the bottle or mix it in water or their favorite cool beverage at any time. For support with digestion or allergy, it is best to take it before breakfast and dinner, undiluted or with a very small amount of water. For other applications the Aloe Vera juice can be taken at any time, 3-4 hours before bedtime. Most consumers begin to sleep better at night after beginning to drink a quality Aloe Vera juice regularly. Yet if consumed right before retiring, the energizing components in the juice can keep some people awake. If diarrhea occurs, reduce the daily amount taken until formed bowel movements return. Most consumers welcome more regularity, yet for sensitive bowels, begin with just a teaspoon of Aloe Vera juice and increase over a 2-3 week period, to the desired amount as the bowels allow. Aloe Vera being 100% safe may be consumed in larger amounts as desired, yet always begin with the suggested amount in the directions on a bottle of juice. Then slowly increase to the desired daily amount.

Because Aloe Vera has a toning effect on the pancreas, which lowers blood sugar, consumers concerned with low blood sugar find taking Aloe Vera with meals the best time. Diabetics on medication also need to begin drinking a small quantity of Aloe Vera juice spread out over the day to avoid unexpected low blood sugar results. Many diabetics have found the Aloe Vera juice helpful in improving their sugar counts while also improving their daily energy throughout the day.

Always begin children on a smaller amount of juice than an adult would drink and gradually increase to the desired daily amount. For most health support, quality Aloe Vera juices can be taken as directed on the bottle. In my clinical observation more is needed when individuals seek to apply the immune support of Aloe Vera. To stimulate the immune system higher quantities do seem to give better results. I have observed tumor reduction with as little as 3 ounces per day of the stronger Whole Leaf juice concentrate when taken daily. Some reports have indicated up to 8 ounces were consumed and spread throughout the day. Aloe Vera is not a cure for any disease yet it seems to allow healing to occur that would normally not be as successful without its use. Important: Do not stop any of your current medications prescribed by a physician. Aloe Vera is considered a food-dietary food supplement and can be added to any health program that your doctor or health practitioner has designed for you. (See caution of use of Aloe Vera for possible sensitivity to Aloe.) *Consumer Beware:* Aloe Vera is a natural blood thinner as is Vitamin E. Stop taking both supplements two weeks before any surgery to avoid a lack of blood clotting ability. Two weeks after surgery, Aloe Vera and Vitamin E can be resumed as tolerated.

FDA Disclaimer:

Aloe Vera is considered a nutritional dietary supplement and has not been tested for health benefits according to the standards set by our government agency called the FDA. It has been approved by our government as a vegetable food additive only and has been regulated for its laxative properties.

Definitions of Aloe Vera products:

- *Aloe Vera Juice-* Made from the inner fillet alone. Even if the label states 99% pure Aloe Vera it can contain as little as 15% Aloe or less at times.
- *Aloe Vera Gel-* Made from the inner fillet to which a thickening agent such as Carrageenan, Xanthan Gum or Irish Moss has been added. It is not the natural thickened property from the plant as one might think. Potency may vary.
- *Whole Leaf Aloe Vera Juice-* Made from the entire leaf including the skin, rind, sap and inner gel. Contains 12% higher solids than the inner gel alone. These solids contain 3-5 times more polysaccharides. Remember, each brand of product will have varying degrees of Aloe Vera content.
- *Whole Leaf Aloe Vera Juice Concentrate-* Made from the entire leaf and does not have any water added if made from an ethical company. Concentrates remove a percentage of natural water from the plant juice without using heat. They contain the highest amounts of solids and polysaccharides **especially Activaloe**.

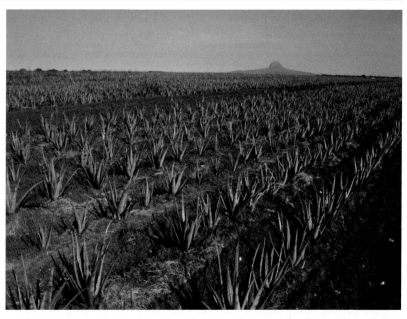

This type could be considered the highest quality Aloe Vera juice. It is best if made from fresh juice, no water added, no sulfites and containing active aloe constituents. Once again, each brand of concentrate product will have varying degrees of Aloe Vera content.

- *200:1 or 400:1 Aloe Vera Juice-* Liquid products that are labeled in this manner are made from powdered Aloe Vera that has been reconstituted commonly with; 1 part Aloe Vera powder to 199 parts of water. It is impossible to concentrate fresh juice to this concentration. This fact makes the ethics of a company claiming this number questionable. Consumers beware! Any liquid Aloe Vera product can be made from powdered Aloe Vera. It is best to look for products that state made from fresh juice, no sulfites and no water added. I have observed more health benefits when using fresh undiluted Aloe Vera products. Unless otherwise stated, the 200:1 will also be made from the inner gel only, supplying limited active ingredients.

- *Fractionally Distilled Aloe Vera-* Consumer beware! Read the labels of all Aloe Vera products. Even though this type of product is labeled Aloe Vera juice, it states on the label, fractionally distilled *from* Aloe Vera. Testing shows no solids are present in this type of Aloe

Vera. It tastes like water because distillation extracts primarily water from the plant juice. This type of Aloe Vera product may contain the volatile mineral sulfur. This would explain why consumers do receive a marginal benefit. The active ingredients in Aloe Vera are primarily located in the 1% solids portion of the plant juice. According to laboratory testing, none of the valuable polysaccharides, amino acids or anti inflammatory elements, (excluding sulfur) etc., are present in this type of juice.

Proper packaging of Aloe Vera Juice for drinking:

Aloe Vera is a nutrient rich vegetable containing vitamins, minerals, enzymes, proteins and healthy lipids. Look for products that are packaged properly, to protect the juice constituents from light damage. Exposure to light may destroy the active constituents of Aloe. Some companies use clear glass or clear plastic that may greatly reduce the nutritional value received by the consumer. Opaque white food grade plastic is considered extremely safe from plastic residue and the best for prevention of nutrient damage. It also keeps the price affordable.

Aloe Vera as a Preventative Health Drink

The people of Mexico and South America have used the Aloe Vera plant known as Sabila, for centuries. Thousands of people, around the globe use this healing plant on a daily basis in their diet to prevent disease. This could be an excellent idea for more people to follow since disease is on the rise in the world.

Scientific research confirms the top 3 diseases of developed countries are diet & lifestyle related:
1.) Cardiovascular Disease
2.) Cancer
3.) Diabetes

In the United States and in the United Kingdom, a person dies from heart disease every 30 seconds. Research confirms that one out of three adults will have Cancer in their life time. In some areas, Diabetes is

31

almost epidemic in certain ethnic groups over the age of 60. The top three diseases of the modern world are Cardiovascular Disease, Cancer and Diabetes. Scientific research confirms that all three are diet and lifestyle related. Although modern medicine can keep an ailing body alive longer in the 21st century, how to actually keep a body vitally healthy and productive has become a challenge to both the individual citizen and the medical community alike. Most physicians are not taught extensive health and nutrition in medical school. Therefore, the individual must take action to educate themselves about restoring health and at the same time working together with their doctors as a team.

With small exceptions, I find modern medicine is focusing on treating disease rather than prevention of disease. Doesn't it make perfect sense to begin more preventative measures in your life? "An ounce of Aloe is better than a pound of cure."

Aloe Vera supports the most important body functions:
- Digestion & Liver function
- Normalize Blood Sugar
- Elimination & Healing function
- Healthy Cholesterol
- Immune & Auto Immune function
- Detox & Bioavailability

Out of both desperation and common sense, people around the world are learning more about health. Many are relying, once again, on time honored herbs and healing traditions of their ancestors, to regain and maintain health. Just imagine feeling better and looking younger even though you've never been older! The ability to reverse ageing has been proven at Tufts University in the Human Nutrition Research Center. The study was conducted over a ten year period, with thousands of doctors and nurses. It showed even after the age of 60, people were able to reverse the aging process, through nutrition and exercise. However, it takes effort! Aloe Vera supports the most important body functions including: digestion and liver function, elimination, healing and immune and auto-immune function.

A clinical observation in support of Aloe Vera for detoxifying the liver from poisonous chemicals:

I met a gentleman by the name of Frank. He had been spraying the toxic asbestos insulation for years before anyone knew how dangerously toxic it was for the body. Thirty years ago he began drinking an ounce of Aloe Vera juice daily. He told me all of the other men working with him spraying asbestos, had died years ago from cancer. Frank said, "No one has ever done a study with asbestos and Aloe Vera, yet I am not going to stop drinking it!"

Russian researchers conducted a study to see if Aloe Vera would increase the body's ability to handle toxic substances. The test was conducted on rabbits. After half of the rabbits were given Aloe Vera for 30 days, all of the test rabbits were given deadly doses of the lethal chemical strychnine. One third of the rabbits given Aloe Vera survived where all of the controls not receiving Aloe Vera died. The study suggests, the natural protective functions of the human body, may be enhanced, by this miracle plant with no potential side effects.

Sources of Harmful Chemicals in our environment:
- Air
- Food
- Water
- Prescription Drugs

Our world's environment is laden with over 4,000 chemicals in the air, food and waterways. Even with the strictest of health regimens, no one can escape all of the contaminants. Chemicals can also come into our body's environment, in the form of prescription drugs. Have you read the drug information on many of the commonly used prescription medications of today? If you dare to read the side effects, you will read about liver toxicity, cancer and even diabetes. Twenty or so other possible life altering side effects may be listed in the smallest print possible. Taking an over the counter (OTC) popular medication like aspirin can greatly weaken the kidney functions of the body. Yet so many people take aspirin compounds that consumers think of it as harmless. Sometimes a persons health state is so poor, they are almost trapped into taking potentially, harmful drugs to keep living. However it is never too late to get healthier. Check with your doctor or pharmacist and make certain you are not taking drugs that you do not need or that may be causing more harm than good.

Drinking Aloe Vera juice everyday could be one of the wisest things you could do to support your health!

Quality Aloe Vera juice helps to cleanse the body of harmful chemicals, no matter where they originate from; pharmaceutical drugs, environmental poisons or even the body's own waste products. Drinking Aloe Vera juice will not interfere with any other medicine you are taking. It is a vegetable juice. Your doctor would not tell you not to drink a vegetable juice would he/she? Drinking Aloe Vera juice every day could be one of the wisest things you could be doing to support your health!

This section has been included to outline health regimens that have greatly helped others and actually reversed the following conditions. Some individuals choose to only drink a quality Aloe Vera juice and judge the results. I encourage you to start with only the juice and then experiment with the dietary and lifestyle improvements. Then add the support nutrients as tolerated. Aloe Vera is not a cure for disease. It helps rebalance ones health to facilitate healing. Purchase the highest quality supplements from health food stores so you can trust the purity and label claims of the products.

Key: (a) = adult dose, i.u. = international units measurement of oils, m.g. = milligrams, EFA = essential fatty acids, NAC = N-Acetyl Cysteine, micelized = liquid oils that are easier to digest, sublingual = liquid to take under the tongue for best absorption, T. = tablespoon which equals 3 teaspoons, 2 T. equals 1 ounce, Ester = type of Vitamin C that absorbs greater so less is needed, fish oil = a source of Vitamin A that is absorbed much more easily than beta carotene, Quality Aloe Vera = Whole Leaf Aloe Vera Concentrate stating no sulfites or water added.

Acne & Skin- Acne consists of skin blemishes and pustules on the face and body. Acne is greatly effected by digestion, glandular health and nutrition. For best results avoid fried foods and sweets. Include more vegetables in the diet. Drink Aloe Vera juice before meals and apply a therapeutic Aloe Vera Skin Gel with no water added, on the skin twice daily to restore the acid pH needed for healthy skin. Apply the Skin Gel after washing the face and body properly. Aloe Vera is an astringent which closes the pores. Apply a moisturizer after the skin gel, to maintain proper protection of the skin and prevent over production of the oil glands. Aloe helps to reverse scarring. Avoid constipation. See the Diet and Candida section.
Support Nutrients: Aloe Vera, protein, Calcium, Magnesium, Zinc-50 mg.(a), B-Complex 50 mg.(a), Vit.A 25,000 IU(fish oil) 1-2 per day(a), Silica, Vit E d-alpha natural type, Vitamin C, Probiotics, fiber and EFA (essential fatty acids), Caprylic Acid. Drink 32-64 oz. of water and expose the body to daily sunshine whenever possible.

Anemia- Anemia is a condition of low red blood cells that can be effected by nutrition, poor digestion, blood loss, a disease and even the environment. Fatigue and headaches are the most common symptoms. Red blood cells are made in the bone marrow, inside our larger bones. Drinking Aloe Vera juice preferably before meals, seems to stimulate the bone marrow production of red blood cells and all lymphocytes, including white blood cells. Cancer patients including leukemia patients have shown great benefit before and during chemotherapy treatments, by drinking the strongest therapeutic Aloe Vera juice. A daily regimen of 2-4 T. before meals is ideal. See Immune System section.

Support Nutrients: Aloe Vera, protein, Vitamin E, C, A, Zinc, minerals, folic acid, B-Complex, B-12 sublingual, liquid liver by Enzymatic Therapy and Iron as needed. *Note: Too much iron is toxic and can be measured in a laboratory blood test. Avoid environments high in EMF, Electro Magnetic Fields. EMF are found emitted by all electrical machines such as beepers, cell phones, clocks, radios, etc.. Especially avoid sleeping in a highly charged EMF environment.*

Allergies- Allergies are caused by unwanted irritants entering into the blood stream from the outside world such as; pollens, chemicals, animal dander, dust and food particles. The allergens enter into the blood stream through weak cell membranes that have microscopic holes. They cause irritation or histamine reactions like sneezing, scratchy nose and throat, irritated eyes, digestive disturbances, asthma, hay fever, rashes and hives, fatigue, migraines, colds, hyperactivity, mental disorders and even fuzzy thinking. Factors that influence allergies, besides heredity weakness, are poor digestion, elimination and colon health, Candida, and nutrition. Drink Aloe Vera juice, 2-8 T., best before meals. Increase to the amount as needed. A quality Aloe Vera juice (No Water Added!) will help stimulate weak digestion always present with allergies. Needed hydrochloric acid levels (HCL), are often low in children as well as adults. Drinking quality Aloe Vera juice encourages HCL to be released in the stomach. It also helps to strengthen the cell wall integrity through collagen support of the cell membrane which may prevent allergens from entering into the blood stream and causing reactions. Avoid constipation. See the Candida, Detox, Leaky Gut and Digestion sections. Some people are very allergic to Garlic, onions and green foods. For many allergy sufferers avoid milk products (not including eggs and butter) and follow the Gluten free diet for 3 weeks in Diet #2. This may help reduce allergies considerably. *Note:* Some individuals with chemical sensitivities feel better using Organically Grown meat and other foodstuffs. Keep a food diary and make a note each day of how you feel to help track your reactions to different foods. Molds present on many foods and in the environment cause reactions that can confuse the allergy investigation. Peel vegetables and fruits before eating or wash with very diluted chlorine bleach or Grapefruit Seed extract found in the healthfood store and rinse well. Allergies improve as ones overall health improves. *Support Nutrients* as tolerated: Aloe Vera,, Vitamin C -3 grams, ester type (a), bioflavonoids, B-Complex, Zinc, minerals, Vitamin E, Probiotics, EFA, and protein. For some individuals an extra digestive supplement may be necessary.

A.D.D.- Attention deficit disorder and **Mental Health** is a growing concern. Children as well as adults can exhibit the symptoms of A.D.D. or Bipolar, restlessness, poor attention span, slow learning abilities and behavior problems (hyperactivity). Poor digestion prevents the absorption of proteins and minerals that are important for mental clarity and the ability to relax. Other factors to consider are allergies and low blood sugar. Avoid eating processed foods, high in sugar and fats. Junk foods contain minimal nutritional content and set the stage for unhealthy behavior. Diet plays a very important role in restoring balance without drug therapy or can help to minimize the use of drug therapy. Drink quality Aloe Vera juice daily, best before meals, 1-2 T.. For young children, look for the products with 100% natural fruit juice added. Avoid artificial coloring in foods and soft drinks with phosphates. This chemical may interfere with mineral absorption from the body. Also avoid chocolate, caffeine and experiment with a gluten free diet for 3 months. See Diet #2 and see Allergy and Candida sections.
Support Nutrients as tolerated: Aloe Vera, protein 3-4 times per

day, free form amino acids or nutritional yeast, minerals, Calcium, Magnesium, Zinc, lecithin, Vitamin E, B-Complex, Vitamin A, EFA, DHA Omega 3 oil, algae, ginko biloba, water, sunshine and exercise.

Arthritis- Arthritis is the inflammation of a joint or joints. Inflammation causes pain in the body. Arthritis has three types; accident injury, rheumatoid and degenerative (osteoarthritis) type. Rheumatoid arthritis has two components, viral and an auto-immune factor. The *anti inflammatory elements* in a strong quality Aloe Vera juice, the *high sulfur* content and the *aid to digestion*, give all three types of Arthritis varying stages of relief. Arthritis due to accident injury or rheumatoid type seems to respond the best to drinking Aloe Vera juice. The degenerative Arthritis is effected greatly by diet and exercise. Reduce all forms of *sugar, caffeine, alcohol* and *heavy meat in the diet, for the best results.* These diet factors may cause a loss of minerals from the body causing more pain. Minerals are important for building strong bones, teeth and providing proper muscle and tendon function. For some individuals, the nightshade vegetable family of tomato (including tomato products), eggplant and potato will cause more symptoms. Citrus fruits may also cause more pain in the joints when eaten. Lack of liver function, infection in the joints of viral or bacterial organisms, excessive copper and nutritional deficiencies are all factors that may contribute to arthritis. Some types of arthritis can be viewed as modern day scurvy. Vitamin C is very important. All forms of Arthritis is preceded by poor digestion. Drink 2-4 T., of Aloe Vera juice before meals. See Diet sections.

Support Nutrients as tolerated: Aloe Vera, Vitamin C -3 grams, ester type (a), bioflavonoids, Cod Liver Oil, alfalfa tablets, Calcium-Magnesium-Zinc, minerals, EFA, B-Complex, B-12 sublingual, lecithin, bee pollen & royal bee jelly, glucosamine sulfate, chondroitin sulfate, MSM, protein from vegetable sources, water, sunshine. Movement such as walking or stretching exercise is very important daily as tolerated.

Asthma- Asthma is defined as an allergic respiratory disease marked by labored breathing, chest constriction and coughing. An old remedy for asthma was to boil some Aloe Vera leaves in a pan of water and carefully breathe the vapor. The properties in drinking Aloe Vera in modern times, including the anti -inflammatory properties, have been very beneficial for all ages with asthmatic conditions. Drink quality Aloe Vera 1-2 T. before each meal or as needed. Follow diet #2 guidelines. See the Candida, Detox and Allergy section. Anti-parasitic support may also be helpful. Keep dairy products (not including eggs and butter) and gluten foods, low in the diet. Avoid constipation. *Support Nutrients as tolerated*: Aloe Vera, Vitamin C, Bioflavonoids, minerals, Glutathione or N-Acetyl-Cysteine, CoQ 10 enzyme, B-15 (pangamic acid), EFA, Vitamin E, Vitamin A (fish oil), B-Complex, Niacin (not timed release), Vitamin D3, Magnesium, Grapefruit Seed Extract, water and sunshine.

Auto Immune (over 80 types) – Lupus, Rheumatoid Arthritis, Multiple Sclerosis, Chronic Fatigue Syndrome, Bowel Disease, Hashimoto (thyroiditis), Diabetes, many Skin Disorders and even mental imbalances may be associated. A simple definition is the body's immune system becomes overactive and begins to destroy its own healthy tissue while increasing inflammation response. These conditions may also relate to viral components, nutritional deficiencies, poor digestion, stress factors and secondary infections. Take quality Aloe Vera 1 – 2 T. before each meal. Avoid constipation. A nutritious diet including orange, yellow and green vegetables with quality proteins is important. Gluten intolerance may be a factor. See diet #1 and #2. Drink good water and exercise. *Support Nutrients:* Aloe Vera, Greens Vegetable Drink, Multiple Vitamin and Mineral, Liquid B12, B-Complex 50 mg. (a), CoQ-10, Essential Fatty Acids, Vitamin E, Vitamin C, NAC or Glutathione, Lecithin, Alpha Lipoic Acid, Probiotics and Liquid Silver.

Bladder Infections and Interstitial Cystitis- Infections show a need for more protein and Vitamin A. If these foods are abundant in the diet then poor digestion is a factor. Bladder, urethra and vaginal infections may also indicate a low immune function. *Note:* If a chronic condition exists in a sexually active person HIV testing is important to rule this factor out. It may also be important to treat the sex partner for a bladder infection even though symptoms may not be present. This is especially important if the infection is reoccurring. Drink a quality Aloe Vera juice daily, 2-4 T., to support digestion and stimulate immune function. Avoid caffeine. See Immune System section. If fever is present consult a physician as needed. If burning sensation take 1/2 tsp of baking soda in water. See Candida. *Support Nutrients:* Aloe Vera, Cod Liver Oil or Vitamin A (50,000 i.u. fish oil)(a), and Goldenseal and Echinacea (10 days), Vitamin C, E, Uva Ursi (herb), NAC, Probiotics, carrot, apple juice and green juices.

Burns- All burns can be serious and should not be treated lightly, particularly beyond second degree burns. Besides the pain and possible scarring, there can be great danger for infection. Medical attention is important. Aloe Vera is excellent for first-aid treatment for sunburn or burns by other means. Aloe Vera stops pain and reduces the chance of infection and scarring, while enhancing the healing process. You can use it first, even if medical treatment may be required later. Apply twice daily to reach the best results with the strongest Whole Leaf Aloe Vera topical skin gel. Placing a liquid quality Aloe Vera juice in a spray bottle will allow application to sensitive areas. *Note:* Preservatives in the products may give some degree of burning initially before relief follows from the Aloe Vera.

> First Degree- skin not broken
> Second Degree- blisters and skin broken
> Third Degree-all layers of skin destroyed and open wound
> Fourth Degree- skin charred

Supportive Nutrients and other: Aloe Vera, multiple vitamin and mineral, protein, EFA, balanced whole foods diet, medical attention as needed.

Cancer & HIV - See Immune System section.

Candida- Candida albicans is the name of a fungal (yeast) organism naturally occurring in the human body. It becomes a health threat when it over grows and travels systemically through the blood stream. A coated tongue (white to brown) referred to as "Thrush" or frequent vaginal infections in women are two common symptoms that show Candida over growth. Factors that influence Candida include antibiotic use, chemotherapy, constipation, eating junk food, poor digestion and a weak immune system. <u>Candida can block absorption of nutrients from our foods and supplements resulting in malabsorption that may complicate any disease conditions.</u> *Candida worsens allergies and is a big factor in many diseases including: Chronic Fatigue, Cancer, Fibromyalgia, HIV(AIDS), and Irritable Bowel Syndrome.* See diet #2 and Detox section. A high protein, low carbohydrate diet with an abundance of vegetables is recommended. Keep sugar and dairy products very low. It is extremely important to keep the bowels regular. Some individuals feel worse when consuming Garlic, onions or Vitamin C until the bowels become more regular. Drink 1-2 T. or more of quality Aloe Vera juice before each meal to encourage regularity, digestion and help stimulate the immune system. *Support Nutrients:* Aloe Vera, free form amino acids, Vitamin A (fish oil), Vitamin C, Vitamin E (micelized), EFA, Probiotics, liquid B-Complex (sublingual), caprylic acid, minerals, Calcium, Magnesium, Zinc, Garlic (as tolerated), CoQ 10 enzyme 30 mg. 2-4 daily, NAC or glutathione, water, exercise, Pau d'Arco, Goldenseal for 7-10 days, Liquid Silver, Green Supplement as tolerated.

Cardiovascular Disease (CVD) & Blood Pressure – CVD, commonly called heart disease is the #1 Killer in the U.S. and U.K... A By-Pass surgeon, Dr. Dean Ornish, M.D., developed an excellent health program reversing blockages that could have led to a heart attack. Low in animal protein, a minimum of 1 oz. of alcohol, high in vegetables and food fiber, along with 45 min. of aerobic exercise daily worked for most. See Diet #1 & #2. Also, a healthy liver is important to process fat soluble vitamins known as anti-oxidants, Vitamins A, E, and EFA's. Plus B, C and garlic are found to be very valuable fighting CVD. Aloe Vera supports digestion, regularity and liver function greatly along with food fiber from beans, fruits and vegetables. Excessive cholesterol is removed in daily bowel movements. Drink quality Aloe Vera, 1-2 T. before meals is best. Research has supported Aloe Vera to lower cholesterol along with fiber in the diet. High potassium rich foods support lowering Blood Pressure as a bonus. *Supportive Nutrients:* Aloe Vera, Vitamin A, C 3,000 mg. and E 200 – 800 i.u. (a), CoQ-10, B-Complex 50 - 100 mg. (a), (fish oil) EFA's 3,000 mg., Calcium & Magnesium Citrate, Greens Supplement (as tolerated), Aged Garlic.

Colds & Flu- There exists thousands of viruses. Viruses are infectious organisms that develop into colds & flu. Doctors cannot treat the cold and flu viruses. Persons must build up a resistance to viruses through health practices. Many people that begin drinking Aloe Vera juice daily report their incidence of colds and flu are reduced greatly. Research has shown Aloe Vera stimulates certain immune functions to reduce viral replication. Take 2-4 T. daily for prevention. When ill, drink 2 tablespoons or more of Aloe Vera juice every 3-4 hours as tolerated. If fever is present drink plenty of fluids, make certain the bowels are regular and consult a physician. Reduce daily stress and get proper rest. See Immune System, Detox and Diet section. Gargling with Aloe Vera Juice has been very soothing for a sore throat. Swallow the juice after the treatment.

Supportive Nutrients: Aloe Vera, Vitamin A, C and E, B-Complex, protein, Zinc, Calcium, Magnesium, NAC, Lacto B. Probiotics, Echinacea, Golden Seal (10 days).

Constipation & Leaky Gut- The body is designed to eliminate waste products through the intestinal tract on a daily basis. In undeveloped countries where people eat a diet without processed foods, high in nutrition, fiber (low gluten) and water, constipation does not exist. Factors needed for regularity include; Calcium, Magnesium, fiber, oil, water, exercise, muscle tone and health of the colon including regular bathroom visits. Whole Leaf Aloe Vera Concentrate juice contains the highest amount of laxative property called anthraquinones without becoming dependent. African Black Aloe products are considered harsh laxatives that may leave the user reliant on it for regularity. Two other laxative herbs that may become almost addictive are Cascara Segrada and Senna. Note: Psyllium fiber may be helpful to some in bulking stool yet for approximately 35% or more of the public it adds to the constipation and bloating problem along with ground flaxseed. Flax may contain sharp particles that damage the microscopic villi of the small intestine. See Allergy, Digestive and Diet #2 Low Gluten sections. Note: For Lazy Bowel, using enemas and or colonic therapy may be methods to encourage evacuation of the bowel without chemicals or laxatives. Daily Greens Drink, Prunes, Figs, Pineapple, Papaya, Apples, Raw Carrots, Celery, Beets and water are helpful.

Supportive Nutrients: Aloe Vera, Vitamin, A, C, E, Magnesium Citrate, Vegetable Oil, Cod Liver Oil, Probiotics, Garlic.

Dental & Oral Hygiene - The health status of the mouth, teeth, tongue and gums, are directly related to the health of the individual. If you are experiencing multiple dental problems then take this as a warning that you need to improve your eating habits including more quality protein, vegetables and more attention to digestion and elimination. Reduce or stop abusive habits such as sugar, alcohol, smoking and or drug abuse. Gargle and drink quality AloeVera Juice. Use a qualityAloe Vera Skin Gel for actually brushing the teeth, tongue and gums. This will make a remarkable improvement with your oral hygiene. Especially helpful with braces. Research has shown very positive support for Aloe Vera decreasing cavities and gum disease. See Candida section if the tongue or gums have a white coat or spots. *Supportive Nutrients:* Aloe Vera, Vitamin C, Bioflavonoids, Vitamin A, B-Complex, minerals, protein, Probiotics.

***Dandruff & Hair Care*-** Flakes on the scalp and more seriously seborrhea dermatitis can both be in the category of dandruff. Emotional traumas, illness, hormonal imbalance and nutritional deficiencies can stimulate dandruff to develop. Uncontrolled dandruff can lead to hair loss and baldness. Dandruff can often be controlled through diet and applying Aloe Vera juice topically to the scalp. A quality Aloe Vera Skin Gel 1-2 tsp., can also be easily applied to the scalp after washing the hair. Drink a quality Whole Leaf Aloe Vera Juice Concentrate and add juice to your shampoo, 1/3 Aloe Vera and 2/3 Shampoo. Wash as normal 2 – 3 times per week. See Diet #2. *Supportive Nutrients:* Aloe Vera, Vitamin A, Vitamin B-Complex 50 mg.(a), Niacin, Vitamin C, Vitamin E, EFA, selenium, Zinc, protein.

***Detoxify & Cleansing*-** Waste products are made daily by every cell of the body. Pollutants are ingested in the air we breath and the water and food that we consume. Sleeplessness, illness and drug abuse (including alcohol & smoking) all create more waste products in the body. People get tired at night because of the toxic build up in the tissues. Sleep allows the body to detoxify. <u>The skin, lymph, lungs,</u>

liver, kidneys, and bowels are channels of detoxification. When the body receives the proper nutrients, water and exercise, a natural process of eliminating toxins takes place and energy and well being is experienced. Unfortunately many people do not give the body what is required to detoxify and the body stores the waste products in the cells and tissues of the body. Symptoms of toxicity are fatigue, fuzzy thinking, bloating, constipation, bad breath, lung congestion, skin disease, headaches, achy joints and illness. To detoxify the body, begin eating more fruits and vegetables as tolerated, approximately 2 cups per day. Reduce junk foods. Eat 50% raw foods and drink 36-48 ounces of good drinking water or vegetable juice daily. Open the body's pores through hot baths, saunas, etc.. Drink a quality Aloe Vera juice 1-2 T., before each meal is best. See Diet and Candida sections.

Supportive Nutrients: Aloe Vera, Burdock Root, Rhubarb Root, Dandelion Root, Ginseng, Chamomile, Slippery Elm, Pau d'Arco, Alfalfa, Fenugreek Tea, Wheat Grass, Algae, Garlic as tolerated, NAC, Vitamin C, Magnesium, multiple vitamin and mineral, Beets, Daikon Radish, fiber, 1-2 T. of olive oil, flax oil, waterolive oil, coconut, flax, fish oil and greens.

Diabetes & Blood Sugar- The pancreas organ is responsible for secreting digestive enzymes and insulin for proper sugar metabolism. Nutritional abuse, weak hereditary factors, a lack of exercise and autoimmune may lead to poor functioning of the pancreas linked to diabetes. It is the 4th cause of death globally and in the U.S. To reverse this disease process, diet, digestion and exercise, all three, play very important roles. Sugars and lipids (fats and oils) are the main dietary abuse categories and important to regulate for longevity. Eat 6 smaller meals daily including; proteins from fish, lean meats along with natural sugars from complex carbohydrates from legumes and low gluten grains. Vegetables including green beans and leafy green vegetables are good while reducing high glycemic ones. Drink 1-2 tsp. of quality Whole Leaf Aloe Vera Concentrate juice before each meal is best. Research shows glucose levels may reduce in just minutes so adjust as needed. Regular meals are absolutely necessary to stabilize blood sugar. Keep meals simple but nutritious. See Diet section. Note: Monitor glucose levels closely.

Supportive Nutrients: Aloe Vera, Chromium Picolinate, Vanadium, minerals, protein 3-4 portions daily, free form amino acids, Nopal Cactus, Vitamin E, B-Complex and water.

Digestive Disorders- Irritable Bowel Syndrome includes all digestive disturbances such as; diverticulitis, Crohn's, celiac sprue, gastritis, constipation, diarrhea, reflux, hiatal hernia, etc.. Most adults, including children, do not secret proper amounts of HCL, hydrochloric acid, into the stomach. Therefore gas, belching and bloating results, with irregular bowel movements as well. The HCL has an acidic pH and is necessary for digesting proteins and minerals from our foods. It also kills parasites and bacterial microorganisms that should not enter the body. Aloe Vera helps maintain a proper acidic balanced environment in the intestines, to prevent overgrowth of fungus conditions such as Candida. Stomach aches can feel like too much acidity is present, yet most often it is due to an HCL deficiency. Drink a quality Aloe Vera juice 1-2 T. before each meal is best. Dietary improvements and restrictions are also important. See Diet #2 for IBS. *Note:* Only 12 % of consumers may truly be too acidic. A test for acidity is to squeeze 1-2 T. of lemon juice or apple cider vinegar into water and drink before meals. If you feel better after this, then drinking Aloe Vera will help greatly. If you receive more stomach upset, then Stomach Plus Aloe Vera is best. Also use Probiotics and include more vegetables and greens in your daily diet. Digestive Enzymes may not be needed with most people if drinking a quality Whole Leaf Aloe Vera Juice Concentrate containing the "yellow sap". See Diet #2.

Supportive Nutrients: Whole Leaf Aloe Vera Concentrate, Probiotics, Fish or Flax Oil, Minerals, Daily Greens (gluten free), Vitamin A, C, E, B, B12, Fiber (gluten grain free), L-Glutamine (as tolerated) and Stomach Plus juice.

Ear Infections- Pain in the ears, sensitivity to cold weather, fever and dizziness can all be symptoms of an ear infection. Factors that may also cause discomfort in the ears are allergies, Candida, wax build up and colds. *Note:* With fevers always consult with a medical physician. Children and adults that swim, surf, have food allergies or frequent colds, more frequently develop ear infections. The need for a strong immune system and a good diet high in protein and Vitamin A is important. Good digestion is required to absorb these nutrients properly into the blood stream for children and adults. A quality Aloe Vera juice supports both digestion, liver functions and immunity. Drink 1-3 ounces of quality Aloe Vera juice daily, best before meals or anytime. See Candida and Immune System section.

Supportive Nutrients: Aloe Vera, protein, Vitamin A(fish oil), C, E, B-Complex, EFA, Calcium, Magnesium, Zinc Lozenger, niacin (a), Probiotics. *Internal Ear drop application of Aloe Vera is safe:* Look for Aloe Vera Ear Drops by Aloe Life or one may dilute a quality therapeutic Whole Leaf Aloe Vera juice product with 50% distilled water. Just 3-5 drops of the dilution into the ear restores the acidic pH, necessary for the healing process and may bring immediate relief of pain or discomfort. Repeat as needed. May also be used for pets.

Energy & Fatigue- Fatigue is experienced by a large percentage of people today. It is a symptom that something is not correct in the body. A healthy body has energy most days without the aid of caffeine. The basic program for creating energy is number one, adequate sleep, 7-9 hours daily. Number two, eat a balanced diet with adequate protein (half your weight in grams), vegetables and grains. Number three, water is very important in sufficient quantities, 24-48 ounces of water daily. Four, for every portion of caffeine add another 8 ounces of water daily. Excessive use of caffeine is more than 3 portions. Using an excessive amount of caffeine beverages may bring about fatigue due to loss of nutrients through the urine. Five, eating excessive sugar or refined carbohydrates, will also bring about fatigue. Six, chemical abuse or even excessive exposure to EMF (Electro Magnetic Fields) can be a factor with fatigue as well. *Note:* Fatigue can be a symptom of a physical or mental state to include; digestive, anemia, pg. 36, blood sugar, pg. 44, high stress, and even Adrenal exhaustion, pg. 37, 51, 53. Seek medical attention as needed coupled with health support. Have regular checkups and blood work to spot deficiencies. Tests can spot anemia, electrolytes, and immunity deficiencies. A urine test for sedimentation rate is also good. Exercise and stretch as tolerated regularly! *Supportive Nutrients:* Aloe Vera, protein, multiple vitamin & minerals,

CoQ 10, EFA, Liver tablets and or Iron, Greens, B[12].

Eye Irritations- Traditional herbal writings have included Aloe Vera as an herbal remedy to reduce eye irritation. Dilute a quality therapeutic Aloe Vera juice product with 50% distilled water and safely apply to the eye area. A slight tingling feeling is natural. Repeat as needed, 1-3 times daily. *Note:* Always consult a medical physician with an eye infection. My children have used this remedy often with eye irritation or "pink eye". Drinking Aloe Vera juice also helps to resolve "floaters" in the eye. See Diabetes sections.
Support Nutrients: Aloe Vera, protein, Vitamin A and C, Rutin, B-Complex, EFA, Ginko Biloba, Daily Greens and Grape Seed Extract.

Eczema & Psoriasis- Both of these skin conditions are characterized by dry scaly patches of skin or small blisters that can cause mild or acute itching, swelling and discomfort. Complementary medicine views skin conditions, as associated with liver and bowel health, digestion weakness, allergies and nutritional deficiencies. Daily sunshine is very important, 5-15 minutes minimum! If this is not possible then purchase a full spectrum light to use indoors on a daily basis. Drink quality Aloe Vera juice 1-2 ounces daily before meals and eat a nutritious diet full of orange, yellow and green vegetables. Special foods include beets, parsley, figs and limes as tolerated. Include more vegetable proteins in the diet without overeating dairy products. See Detox, Allergy and Digestion sections. Exercise daily.*Supportive Nutrients:* Aloe Vera, Cod Liver oil or Vitamin A(fish oil), liquid liver, B-Complex, Vitamin E, EFA, water, NAC or Glutathione, minerals, Milk Thistle, lecithin and enzymes.

Fertility- Glandular health is paramount for fertility to be successful. When the liver is not processing fat soluble vitamins, such as Vitamin E and A efficiently, the result can be low hormone production. Drinking a good quality Aloe Vera juice 1-2 T. before meals, for 3-6 months can encourage the liver as well as the thyroid and sex glands to work more effectively. Vitamin E is also very important. Eat a nutritious diet with adequate protein, moderate exercise with good daily water consumption. See Diet section. Note: Check body temperature and if below 98.6 take a thyroid nutritional supplement,

as directed on the bottle, until it rises.
Supportive Nutrients: Aloe Vera, Vitamin E (400 mg. d-alpha tocopherol), wheat germ oil, kelp, Zinc, Nutritional Thyroid as needed, multiple vitamin and mineral, water and sunshine, 10-20 minutes daily.

Fibromyalgia- Termed by many as a disease of the 90's, fibromyalgia seems to be a combination of several health imbalances including, digestion, thyroid, Candida and perhaps for some a viral component accompanied by major nutritional deficiencies. Drinking the strongest quality Aloe Vera juice 1-8 ounces daily, supports all of the potential factors. Vitamins and minerals in the diet are extremely important. See Candida section and Diet #2.
Supportive Nutrients: Aloe Vera, B-12 sublingual (1,000 iu)(a), Folic Acid, EFA, Vitamin A (fish oil), Caprylic Acid, Probiotics, Nutritional Thyroid, Vitamin E, Magnesium citrate 800mg.(a), Calcium citrate 1000 mg. (a), CoQ 10-30 mg. 1-3 daily.

Frostbite- Apply a quality Aloe Vera Skin Gel to the affected area at least twice daily. *Supportive Nutrients:* Aloe Vera, protein, multiple vitamin and mineral including Vitamin E and B-Complex, Cod Liver Oil.

Gallbladder & Fat Digestion- Bile is a digestive substance that is made in the liver and stored in the gallbladder. When fat and oil called lipids, and fat soluble vitamins A, E, D, and K are consumed in the diet, bile is suppose to be excreted into the small intestines to aid in fat digestion. The high sulfur in Aloe Vera seems to purge the bile duct from the liver allowing bile to flow freely. Aloe Vera Juice 1-2 T. before meals, aids in more complete fat digestion and decreases the pain in the gallbladder and stomach. A balanced diet, exercise and drinking water are all very important steps to keeping the glands of the body functioning better. A gallbladder flush of apple juice and fresh squeezed lemon juice upon rising is very tonifying.
Supportive Nutrients: Aloe Vera, B-Complex, Lecithin, Probiotics, digestive supplement including bile extract, Vitamin A, E, C.

Headaches- Headaches including migraines are a very important signal from the body that something is not functioning correctly. Instead of learning which aspirin like compound lessens a headache faster, why not do some detective work to find out why you have a headache to begin with?

1.) Headaches may come from trauma to the head, pressure from a certain hairstyle, tension in the back and neck.
2.) Poor Digestion & Elimination.
3.) Allergy.
4.) Emotional Upset or Stress.
5.) Anemia from lack of protein, iron, folic acid or B12. (Unbalanced Diet) Laboratory tests can detect certain nutritional deficiencies but not all.
6.) Low Blood Sugar from excessive caffeine, sugar, fried foods, viral infections and possible Diabetic symptoms.
7.) Women's Menses & Hormone Imbalances.
8.) Organic origin needing medical diagnostic work to rule out a rare tumor, etc.
9.) High Blood Pressure.

Aloe Vera taken 1-2 T. daily before meals can reduce the frequency of headaches greatly. Eat 3-6 meals daily. Avoid foods that trigger headaches such as chocolate, coffee, MSG seasoning, cheese (a mold containing food). Keep the bowels regular. See Diet #2 and the Anemia, Candida, Detox and Allergy sections.
Supportive Nutrients: Aloe Vera, EFA, Zinc, protein, Chromium Picolinate, Appropriate Iron, B-Complex (hypo allergenic), free form amino acids, COQ 10.

Hemorrhoids- All tissue structural weakness such as hemorrhoids, have similar deficiencies. Aloe Vera helps build collagen strength to reduce hemorrhoids, bleeding gums, nosebleeds and varicose veins. Drink 1-2 T. of quality Aloe Vera juice before meals. Apply a quality Aloe Vera Skin Gel directly on the hemorrhoids or area of concern. Aloe Vera Skin Gel has also been very helpful with Vaginal dryness.
Supportive Nutrients: Aloe Vera, Vitamin C, Bioflavonoids, EFA, Vitamin E, protein, minerals.

Hepatitis & Liver Disorders- Liver disorders, including the viral condition Hepatitis, effects not only the liver but the entire health potential of the body. Liver damage can result from alcoholism, heavy sugar consumption, poor diet, drug or chemical ingestion (pollutants and even prescription drugs), being overweight and viral infections or exposure to toxic substances. Recently a link between tattoos and hepatitis has been presented as a potential risk for getting hepatitis. The list of ways to contract this potential life threatening virus is also I.V. drug abuse, unclean sex practices and tainted water or food. Essential for recovery and maintenance is a healthy balanced diet. No fried foods. *See Diet section.* Keep the bowels regular. Drink 1-2 T. of quality Aloe Vera before meals. I have worked with many individuals that feel exceptionally well by choosing a health program to follow. Viruses can be put in remission, including Hepatitis C. *Supportive Nutrients:* Aloe Vera, protein, minerals, Vitamin C, (3-12 grams), Bioflavonoids, EFA, Liquid Liver Extract, Glutathione or NAC, Selenium, B-Complex, herb- Milk Thistle, Vitamin E, Probiotics, Digestive Enzymes, lecithin, Nutritional Yeast, B15.

Herpes & Shingles- The viruses that cause Herpes and Shingles are closely related. They are from a family of viruses that cause five different viral conditions in the body including Herpes I & II, Shingles, Chicken Pox and Mononucleosis. Most often these viruses will remain dormant and will not be contagious. However, these viruses become activated when the body's immune system is weakened. This may come from mental or physical stress, disease or sickness, extreme weather conditions like too much sun and lastly, certain irritating foods. Fatigue, headaches, irritability, fuzzy thinking, flu like symptoms, slight fever, skin outbreaks including cold sores are the most common symptoms of the viruses becoming active. <u>Some individuals experience only the inner symptoms without external skin outbreaks.</u> The skin lesions, like tiny blisters, are very transferable, even before they are visible. Eye contact may lead to blindness. Sexual transmission is also very easy during an outbreak. Keeping the virus dormant through health measures is highly recommended. Drink quality Aloe Vera juice before meals, 1-4 oz. daily is best. Avoid citrus, spicy foods, fried foods, chocolate, ice cream and caffeine. Eat a healthy diet with an emphasis on lean meats, eggs, fish and vegetables. Limit your intake of carbohydrate foods that are rich in the amino acid called Arginine. Lysine, a helpful amino acid on the other hand, gives balance to viral conditions. Topical treatment includes a quality Aloe Vera Skin Gel with Vitamin E. Also add lemon balm if available. Topical application stops the pain and speeds the healing. *Supportive Nutrients:* Aloe Vera, Lysine 400 mg. daily and increase to 1200 mg. with an out break, Vitamin C with Bioflavonoids, 1-10 grams, B-Complex 50 mg., B-12 sublingual, Probiotics with Bifidus, Vitamin E 400-1200 mg. (a), Zinc Citrate 20-50 mg. (a), lecithin, NAC, Chromium Picolinate, olive leaf and Red Marine Algae.

Insomnia- Insomnia is a difficulty in falling asleep and in staying asleep. Minerals are essential for the proper functioning of the muscles in the body and actually help people feel more relaxed to sleep well. One way to increase the amount of minerals in your body is with your diet. Eat more green and orange vegetables, raw nuts and seeds, beans including tofu and wholegrains as tolerated. Dairy products are a secondary food source for minerals because some people are allergic to dairy products and they contain limited mineral value. Dairy also does not digest as easily for many people. Some individuals only need to improve the absorption of minerals they are already receiving in their diet, to sleep through the night. Drinking Aloe Vera 1-2 T. before meals increases natural HCL (hydrochloric acid) flow into the stomach. The HCL is essential for mineral digestion and absorption. Avoid excessive caffeine including chocolate. You may wish to keep a diary before bedtime to help purge the daily thoughts and concerns. Take your Calcium, Magnesium and herbal supplements before bedtime. *Supportive Nutrients:* Aloe Vera, Calcium, Magnesium, Zinc, protein, Vitamin A, B-Complex, Vitamin E, Herbs- Chamomile, Hops, Valerian and Passionflower. Melatonin is best used if other means do not help. Daily exercise is very valuable.

Immune System- The Immune System is designed to protect the body from all invading organisms whether it be externally in a wound or to prevent illness. Factors that influence the immune system function besides heredity weakness is diet, stress, drug abuse including smoking and alcohol, exercise and the environment. A weakened area of the body becomes diseased. Disease needs the opportunity to develop. Low immune function often manifest itself with frequent colds, chronic fatigue, allergies, etc. before cancer or other diseases finally develop. The activity of the Immune System can be measured in a blood test that shows how efficient the different levels of immunity register. Infections from viral, bacterial, fungal and allergies stimulate the immune system to activate and keep the body well. Quality Aloe Vera stimulates part of the immune system called macrophage, pgs. 9, 13, 14. When properly stimulated, the macrophages are powerful cells that demonstrate phagocytosis by gobbling up invaders in the blood stream. Much like little pac men ingesting garbage. The Aloe Vera research shows the polysaccharides in Aloe to be primarily responsible for this immune response. Scientists have proven significant anti viral effects from Aloe Vera application with Cancer, Epstein Barr, Herpes, Shingles, HIV, Flu and Measles. Tumor reduction has been observed with the strongest quality Aloe Vera products using 3-8 ounces daily. It is best to begin with a small amount then increase as tolerated. Take in divided does before meals. Results are dose dependent. Caution: If diarrhea results reduce the daily amount of Aloe Vera. See Candida, Digestion, Detox and Diet sections.

Supportive Nutrients: Whole Leaf Aloe Juice Concentrate (Activaloe), Vitamin C (ester type, 3-12 grams), Bioflavonoids, Vitamin A (fish oil, 10,000 1-3 daily), Vitamin E (400 i.u.) (Avoid Vitamin E in larger amounts with hormone sensitive cancer such as breast or prostate cancers), N-Acetyl-Cysteine 500 mg. 1-4 daily or Glutathione, Single cell Algae, minerals, EFA, "Super Oxide Dismutase (S.O.D.), Wheatgrass.

Leaky Gut- The large intestine or gut is approximately 8 feet long. The small intestines are approximately 13 feet in length giving a total of 22 or more feet of intestines in the body. Through years of having intestinal problems including constipation, parasites, Candida overgrowth and even scarring of the intestinal wall with IBS, structural weakness may occur. Bowel disease (See Diet #2) damages the intestinal wall and villi called Leaky Gut. This condition may allow waste products called toxins to leave the intestines and enter into the body tissues. Aloe Vera speeds healing of wounds on the outside of the body as well

as mending the gut on the inside. Drink 1-2 T. before each meal is best. See Diet, Detox, Digestive and the Candida section.
Supportive Nutrients: Aloe Vera, Probiotics, EFA and minerals.

Leg Cramps- Cramps are spasms or an involuntary contraction of a muscle in the leg or foot that can be very painful. They occur commonly at night and more frequently in the elderly, the young and persons with arteriosclerosis. Besides blood circulation, digestion is a major factor along with deficiencies of Calcium, Magnesium, Potassium and Folic Acid. Take Aloe Vera 1-2 T. before meals to encourage HCL production in the stomach that helps to digest and absorb minerals out of your food. "Restless Foot" can be included in this category. See Diet section.
Supportive Nutrients: Aloe Vera, B-Complex, Vitamin E (400-1000 mg.), Calcium Citrate, Magnesium Citrate (800 mg.), EFA, Multiple Digestive Enzyme, Water, Folic Acid, Potassium.

Longevity & Anti-Aging- The body has many systems including:
1.) The Cardiovascular System includes the heart, lungs, veins and arteries.
2.) The Muscular skeletal system with both the bones and muscular components.
3.) The Nervous system which sends messages to the other systems to perform their daily work.
4.) Lymphatic and Immune systems are essential for ridding the body of waste and fighting infections.
5.) The Digestive System provides the body with nutritional building components for every cell.
6.) The Glandular and the Endocrine systems run the growth and development of the body.

We are only as healthy as our weakest link. Research points to the glands as maintaining virility, stamina and longevity. Tufts University found through regular exercise, a nutritious diet and Vitamin E, the study participants were able to reverse aging even after the age of 60. Animal studies on longevity showed eating 3-6 smaller meals instead of 2 or 3 large meals extended the life of the test animals significantly. New Aloe Vera research has confirmed that through daily consumption of Aloe Vera the animals drinking the juice daily showed a 25% life

extension. See Diet, Detox and Digestion sections.
Supportive Nutrients: Aloe Vera, Vitamin E, Vitamin A, Vitamin C, glandular extracts, amino acids, Chromium Picolinate, Ginseng, balanced whole foods diet, Daily Greens, water, exercise, rest, healthy sun exposure and companionship.

Rashes- All skin conditions including rashes, relate to digestion, the health of the liver, proper nutrition and glandular balance. Drink a quality Aloe Vera juice daily and apply a quality Aloe Vera Skin Gel on the skin as tolerated. Always do a skin patch test on a small area to make certain no allergy to Aloe Vera exists. You may need a skin lotion following the topical application of Aloe Vera for very dry skin types. Aloe has been very effective for baby rash and any other skin abnormality. Aloe Vera has given pain relief and reduced scarring with Poison Oak, Poison Ivy and Chicken Pox. See Detoxify.
Supportive Nutrients: Aloe Vera, Vitamin A or Cod Liver Oil, Vitamin E, B-Complex, EFA, Calcium, Magnesium, Zinc and Daily Greens.

Sinusitis - Sinusitus is the inflammation of the sinus membrane. See Diet, Allergy and Candida section. Irrigate carefully into the nose with Aloe Vera juice along with liquid Golden Seal and Echinacea added. Close one nostril and snort liquid off of a spoon. Lay down on your back to allow liquid to drain into the nasal cavities. Consult a physician with infection or fever.

Staph Infections- Healthy skin must maintain an acidic pH. Many soaps and some lotions create an alkaline pH. This coupled with an imbalance in the diet can set the stage for frequent staff infections of the skin. See Diet section. Drink a quality therapeutic Aloe Vera before each meal, 1-2 T. Eating regular nutritious meals is extremely important. Avoid sugar and junk foods. See Candida.
Supportive Nutrients: Aloe Vera, Cod liver oil or Vitamin A (fish oil), B-Complex, protein, dark green and yellow vegetables, water.

Sores & Wounds- People who bruise easily, do not heal in a reasonable time or develop ulcers or wounds on the arms or legs, need to improve their diet. Circulation and immune function are also factors. Drink Aloe Vera juice 1-2 T., before meals. See Diet sections. Exercise or stretching as tolerated is important to stimulate the pancreas to metabolize carbohydrate sugars and improve circulation. Apply a thin layer of Aloe Vera Skin Gel to the wound 3-4 times per week. (See page 17 & 44.) Many find Aloe Life Skin Gel also reverses scars. *Supportive Nutrients:* Aloe Vera, Vitamin E, Chromium Picolinate, EFA, Vitamin C, Bioflavonoids, protein, alfalfa or green drink, Vitamin A and Zinc. Drink sufficient amounts of water daily.

Ulcers (stomach) & Abscess- An internal wound, ulcer or abscess can develop into a very serious health condition if untreated. Many individuals have found Aloe Vera taken before or during a meal reduces pain and speeds healing of an ulcer or internal wound. It is not necessary to stop any medication one might be taking. Aloe Vera can be added to any program. I have found most ulcer patients lack proper HCL to digest and absorb minerals from foods. The Aloe helps balance stomach acids, reduce pain and speeds healing. Even in advanced cases. See Diet #2. Eat 6 small meals daily. Chew your food extremely well or blend in a blender before swallowing. Avoid alcohol and irritants.
Supportive Nutrients: Aloe Vera, EFA, Vitamin A (fish oil), multiple vitamin and mineral, Probiotics, protein.

Diet #1 Daily Regimen Foods For Health
Protein: *3-4 servings-* Eat a variety of protein foods to include: eggs, beans all types including lentils, lean meats; fish, seafoods, chicken, lamb, turkey, only occasionally well cooked-beef or pork, cottage cheese, milk, yogurt, cheeses in moderation, raw nuts & seeds, bean sprouts (fresh), tofu & soy products.

Fruits: *Great for desserts!* Eat all types in season as tolerated. To receive the greatest nutritional value from fruits, eat fresh fruits in season first, frozen second and lastly canned. Drinking too much fruit juice or eating large quantities of fruits can cause a drop in blood sugar, similar to over eating of refined sugar products. It is best to eat whole fruits including melons in moderation.

Vegetables: *3-11 servings-* Eat a variety of steamed vegetables as tolerated. 50% raw as tolerated. Include a variety of dark green, yellow and orange vegetables to include; carrots, squash, yams, potatoes, broccoli, green beans, cabbage, dark green lettuce, radishes including diakon type, tomato, Chinese peas, cucumber, turnips, rutabagas, parsley, chard, all other greens, beets, avocado. ***Grains:*** Rice all types including white & brown, grains including; oats, wheat, barley, rye, millet, etc., breads & pasta all types in moderation. Note: Whole grains like brown rice and whole wheat, contain more food value than refined grains like white rice and white flour products. However, some adults and children are allergic to whole grains (including oats) and feel better eating white rice, quinoa, millet, and other low gluten grains occasionally. See Diet #2.

Fats & Oils: *Use daily in moderation.* Olive oil, sesame oil, canola & other vegetable oils, butter. Margarine and other hydrogenated fats and oils are not recommended. Keep fried foods at a minimum. Store all fats & oils in the refrigerator.

Seasonings: *Use to enhance the enjoyment of food and health support.* Salt in moderation, black & white pepper, red pepper, soy sauce, herbs, onions, Garlic, scallions, chives, parsley, dulse, kelp, etc.

Beverages: Water 32 oz or more, vegetable juice, fruit juice, herbal teas, blender drinks. Drink coffee and black teas in moderation. *It is best to drink liquids between meals. Avoid ice cold beverages at* *mealtimes. Milk is a meal in itself. Keep water or a small amount of other beverage to a minimum with meals not to dilute normal digestive enzymes that are naturally secreted into the foods. Warm liquids are better at mealtimes such as herb teas, black tea, or coffee. Fruit juices are best diluted with water to avoid drinking a concentrated form of fruit sugar for children and adults. Sodas are not a health drink and are best thought of as a dessert to be consumed in moderation if at all. Many adults and children are allergic to cow's milk seek alternatives.*

Snacks: Look to snacks as a nutrition break. There are many healthy snacks that will provide energy and help maintain blood sugar levels. Fresh fruit, cheese slices, raw nuts & seeds, lean meats, hard boiled eggs, yogurt, cottage cheese and fruit, vegetable sticks with or without dressing, fruit juice, popsicles, popcorn. Keep desserts and refined sugary and junk foods low in the diet. 1-2 per week with perhaps a few healthier cookies, etc. throughout the week.

Diet #2 Regenerative Regimen
1.) Yeast Free Candida, 2.) Low Blood Sugar 3.) Herpes 4.) Irritable Bowel Syndrome Diet (IBS) /Gluten Free 5.) Allergies 6.) Chronic Fatigue Syndrome (CFS) [Note: Avoid nuts and seeds with Herpes.]

Protein: *3-6 servings-* Fish & seafood, eggs, lean meats; chicken, beef, turkey, lamb, raw cashews, raw seeds (ground as needed); sunflower seeds, pumpkin seeds, sesame seeds, bean sprouts, egg or other protein powder. Minimize starch vegetables like corn & peas. Keep potatoes, pastas and dairy products low in #2 diet. **IBS Avoid:** Most regular or whole grain pasta, soft cheeses, milk, ice cream and candy. Search for fermented cottage cheese and Greek yogurt as tolerated. 50% of people are cow milk intolerant. Chemicals on processed meats and foods can cause reactions so eat organically grown and fresh when possible. Allergies can cause reactions to chicken, turkey, leafy greens, garlic and onions so review Candida and Detox sections.

Fruits: Eat on a limited basis only as tolerated. Peeled fruits are best to avoid molds. Citrus fruits, are not tolerated by many people in this category. This may be due to the citric acid present. High fruit consumption is not recommended because it has fructose that willencourage yeast to grow and microscopic molds that can upset Candida and IBS. Best to not drink fruit juices.

Vegetables: 3-11 servings per day (2-4 cups)- All vegetables raw and cooked as tolerated, including a variety of dark greens, dark yellow or orange vegetables. To include; carrots, squash, yams, red potato best, green beans, green and red cabbage, dark green lettuce, radishes including diakon type, tomato, Chinese peas, cucumber, avocado, turnips, rutabagas, parsley, chard, all greens, beets and beet tops. *Grains: Keep grains and carbohydrates lower in this diet for all programs until feeling more energy with less symptoms. 1-3 servings of grains to include; all grains on Diet #1 as tolerated.* **IBS to include:** flourless breads, white rice, millet, quinoa, cornflakes, corn meal including corn tortillas, corn chips and polenta, spelt flour and spelt products, white rice flour. *Avoid:* fruit juices, coffee, brown rice, wheat, oats, rye, all regular pastas, flour tortillas, regular potatoes, all regular sweet breads & cookies, regular bread products, pizza, macaroni, etc.. Dark greens may cause symptoms with IBS. Also avoid capsulated and pearled supplements. Best to use powdered, liquid or tableted supplements. Avoid psyllium and flax seed products and concentrate on fiber from your raw vegetables including peeled beets, carrots and apples.

*Fat & Oils: daily-*canola oil, sesame oil, olive oil, or butter. *Supplements as desired;* flaxseed oil, Cod Liver Oil, lecithin, borage oil, black current seed oils. Avoid: Margarine and other hydrogenated fats and oils, fried foods and chips in excess.

Seasonings: Use herbs and seasonings as desired and tolerated . Many people are sensitive to onions, Garlic, leafy herbs because of molds and will experience sick symptoms with use.

Beverages: Water is the best beverage. Avoid herb teas because of natural molds. Black tea seems to be tolerated best if caffeine is desired. Coffee is not tolerated with many regenerative programs especially IBS. Keep all caffeine lower in the diet to feel your best.

Snacks: Best to keep in between meal snacks like mini meals. Hard boiled eggs, lean meats, tuna, cottage cheese and yogurt as tolerated, small amount of fruit as tolerated, popcorn as tolerated, corn chips, raw cashews or seeds as tolerated, vegetable sticks with or without salad dressing, etc.. Keep sweets very low to feel your best.

Diet Tips: 1.) Keep a food diary and make a note of how you feel each day. 2.) If after eating green colored foods like broccoli, green beans or a green supplement, you feel symptoms, avoid greens for one week and see if the symptoms stop. Phenol is a natural chemical present in green foods. Some individuals are sensitive to green foods and feel better leaving them out of their diet. 3.) All people have similarities and differences. Eat the foods that help you feel energetic and well regardless of what you read. Stop eating foods that make you feel sick or experience symptoms even if other people eat them. 4.) Some foods have been mislabeled and state gluten free when in fact they are not free of glutenous properties. 5.) Sugar addiction or any other substance addiction can be very dangerous if not controlled. Seek professional help or possibly a 12 step program in your area. 6.) When it seems like some days you tolerate a food and at other times it makes you sick, this may relate to how much natural *molds* or the *chemical* content of a given food. 7.) If your health condition worsens it is time to review your health program. You may be experiencing a temporary viral condition especially if you feel feverish. For some it may be Candida or another factor stressing your immune system. Experiment with safe non toxic supplements and a healthier diet. Seek a health professional to give you more direction who is familiar with your symptoms. Get some form of exercise started. Do your best and bless the rest!

Whether any of us like it or not human beings need nourishment to survive. Tomorrow is a new day! For some people along with diet and supplement support psychological counseling or group support is very important in getting well and staying well. Don't give up! It is never too late to get healthier!

Diet #3 Detoxification Regimen-Reverse Aging & Disease

1.) *No one cleansing diet is right for all people.* Always consult with a physician or naturopath before beginning a cleansing and detoxification program. This is especially important if you have been under the care of a medical professional and might have multiple health challenges.
2.) *Begin eating 2-4 cups of fruits and vegetables in the daily diet.* 50% raw as tolerated. Chew all of your food well. Many people

begin feeling better by just spending more time chewing their foods. This step will begin the detoxification of the body or in other words eliminating waste from the body. Normal reaction are increase bowel movements, intestinal gas with varying degrees of flu like symptoms. Examples: Headache, nausea, achy joints and stomach bloat. These symptoms will gradually subside.

3.) *Drink 24-48 ounces of good water daily.* Water makes up 75% of the body mass. The glands of the body and lymphatic systems work properly when sufficient amounts of water are consumed. Best to drink in between meals.

4.) *Fasting one day per week allows the body to achieve deeper tissue cleansing.* Fasting is going without eating solid foods. Drinking water and or vegetable juices during the fast is important. Squeezing lemon or lime and Aloe Vera juice in the water adds electrolytes. Fasting for one to seven days is generally looked at as very safe yet a longer fast is best accomplished with the supervision of a health practitioner. Jesus fasted for 40 days and 40 nights to clear his thinking. This is too long for most people to endure. However the body only needs air to breath and water to keep the body alive during short fasting. Drinking diluted juices, herb teas and warm vegetable broth can help fasting be more successful. *Note: If you have low blood sugar or a diabetes condition it is best not to fast. If you begin to feel extremely uncomfortable during your fast begin to eat vegetables and fruits and resume your regular diet.*

5.) *Avoid:* dairy products (during detoxification), junk food, smoking, alcohol and sugar. Roasted nuts, hydrogenated, rancid and excessive fats and oils in the diet will speed up the aging process.

6.) *The bowels must move daily and completely, to reach good detoxification of the body's tissues.* Learn as much as you can about digestion and the health of the colon. *Note:* Fiber plays an important role and is found abundantly in fruits, vegetables and whole grains. Books are available that teach bowel cleansing. Supplements especially Aloe Vera products, Probiotics, wheat grass, alfalfa, Garlic and algae supplements are very helpful for cleaning the bowel. Enemas can also be very effective with lazy bowels both warm water and coffee type. See No. 2 pamphlet for directions. See the longevity and anti aging section for supplements.

7.) *Exercise is absolutely needed in some form.* By moving the body everyday it allows the lymphatic and glandular system to function properly. Move at your own pace and increase your movement as your body allows. Begin 5-10 minutes daily and increase to 30-45 minutes. **Walking in cold water** knee deep can be very stimulating for the circulation and rejuvenating as well. Be safe and wear shoes to avoid glass or etc.

8.) *Breathing fresh air regularly and deeply actually helps to detoxify impurities out of the blood through the lungs.* Viruses cannot live in an oxygenated environment. Remind yourself to breath during the day. Open your windows and buy indoor plants to oxygenate your house if you cannot get outdoors often. Do your best to create a healthy, chemical free environment where you work and live.

9.) *Encourage the Skin to open the pores and stimulate the lymph system to function properly which in turn eliminates waste products from the body.* The skin is the largest eliminating organ of the body. The lymph system exists in every inch of the skin.

   Skin Brushing before a bath or shower regenerates the skin, opens pores and stimulates the lymphatics which expels waste. **Brisk towel drying** after bathing is also very good. **Hot baths** with either a cup of real apple cider vinegar or 1/2 cup of Aloe Vera juice encourages the pores of the skin to detoxify. This has been found to reduce deep pain in the body. **Saunas** are also good. **Therapeutic massage** is the most passive and enjoyable way to help detoxify the body. You can choose to have a trained technician give you a full body massage or learn to do foot massage on yourself. It's been told that the comedian Bob Hope got a massage every day. Maybe that is why he could laugh so much. This method of healing yourself feels good while improving your health.

10.) *Begin each day with meditation or prayer giving thanks and blessings for the day that lies before you.* Make an effort to live 80% healthy with 20% flexibility and you will enjoy the outcome. Health is truly our greatest wealth!

Date: *Foods Eaten*   *Symptom or How You Felt*

Breakfast

Lunch

Dinner

Other:

References for Supplements

1. *Aloe Vera* – Aloe Life International Inc., Higher Nature Ltd. U.K..
2. *Essential Fatty Acids (EFA), Cod Liver Oil* – Nordic Naturals, Flora
3. *Probiotics (Probiotics)* – Dr. Ohirra's, Jarrow, Flora
4. *Vitamin C (Ester Type or other)* – Solgar, Natrol
5. *Vitamin E (d-alpha and mixed), Multiple Vitamin and Mineral* – Aloe Life International Inc, Solgar, Source Naturals
6. *Minerals* – Solgar, Blue Bonnet, Country Life
7. *Herbal Extracts* – Herb Pharm, Aloe Life International Inc.
8. *Glutathione, N-Acetyl-Cysteine* – Jarrow, Solgar
9. *Digestive Enzymes* – Solary, Jarrow, Flora
10. *Gluten Free Greens & Fiber* - Aloe Life International Inc.

Recent Research

Far More Than a Remarkable Folk Medicine: Aloe Vera and A. arborescens, 2019, Yagi, Akira PhD, LAP LAMBERT Academic Publishing, ISBN: 978-613-9-47149-2. Book (75 pages) cover scientific research primarily in Japan and USA, 14 chapters highlighting the value these Aloes have on Immunity, Autoimmunity, Diabetes, Dentistry, Chronic Fatigue, Gut Health, Wound Healing and more.

1.) *Aloe Vera - A Scientific Approach*, 1997, Robert H. Davis, PHD

2.) *The Health and Medical Use of Aloe Vera,* 1996, Lawrence G. Plaskett, Ph.D.

3.) *Rodales's Illustrated Encyclopedia of HERBS*, 1987, Rodale Press

4.) *The Ancient Egyptian Medicine Plant*, 1982, Max B. Skousen

5.) *Nutrition Almanac,* 1984, Nutrition Search, Inc., Kirschmann

6.) *Cancer Facts & Figures-1999*, American Cancer Society

7.) *"Isolation of a Stimulatory System in an Aloe Extract"*, 1991, Davis RH, Parker WL, Sampson RT, Murdoch DP, J Am Podiatr Med Ass 81 (9); 473-478.

8.) *"Aloecin A, an Active Substance of Aloe Arborescens Miller as Immunomodulator"*, 1993, Imanishi, K.

9.) *"Immune Enhancing Effects of Aloe"*, 1992, Pittman JC, M.D., Health Conscious 13 (1); 28-30.

10.) *"Nitric Oxide Production by Chicken Macrophages Activated by Acemannan"* (polysaccharides), 1995, Karaca K, Sharma JM, Nordgren R, Int. J. Immuno Pharmacol. 17(3); 183-188.

11.) *"Studies on the Effect of Acemannan (polysaccharides) on Retrovirus Infections; Clinical Stabilization of Feline Virus-Infected Cats"*, 1991, Sheets, ma et al., Mol. Biother, 3; 41-45

12.) *"Effect of Aloe Extract on Peripheral Phagocytosis in Adult Bronchial Asthma"*, 1985, Shida T, Yagi A, Nishimura H, Nishioka I, Planta Med., 273-275.

13.) *"Mise en evidence et etude proprietes immuno-stimulantes dium extrait isole et partiellement purifie a partir dialoe vahombe"*, 1979, Solar S. et al., Archives de l'Institut Pasteur de Madagascar 47; 9-39.

14.) *"Effects of low molecular Constituents from Aloe Vera Gel on oxidative metabolism and cytotoxic and bacterial activities of human neutrophils"*, 1990, ët Hart LA, Nibbering PH, Van Den Barselaar MT, Van Dijk H, Van Den Berg AJ, Labadie RP, Int. J. Immuno-Pharmacol 12 (4); 427-434.

15.) *"Immunoreactive Lectins in Leaf Gel from Aloe barbadensis Miller"*, 1993, Winters WD, Phytotherapy Res. 7; 523-525.

16.) *" Effect of Amino Acids in Aloe Extract on Phagocytosis by periperal neutrophils in Adult Bronchial Asthma"*, 1987, Yagi A, Jpn J. Allergol. 36 (12); 1094-1101.

17.) *"Aloe Vera Improves Wound Healing and Reduces Inflammation in Diabetes"*, 1987, Davis RH, Pennsylvania Academy of Science 61: 84.

18.) *"Isolation and Hypoglcemic Activity of Arborans A and B, Glycans of Aloe Arborescens Var. Natalensis Leaves"*, 1986, Hikino H, Takahaski M, Murakami L, Konno C, International Journal of Crude Drug Research 24: 183.

19.) *"Anti-Inflammatory and Wound Healing Activity of a Growth Substance in Aloe Vera"*, 1994, Davis RH, DiDonato JJ, Hartman GM, Haas RC, Journal of the American Podiatric Medical Association, 39-51.

20). *"Clinical Evaluation of Full Thickness Wounds with Tunneling and Stage I-IV Wounds:* 100% Resolution with 24 Patients Using PhytoDerm Wound Gel and Improved Wound Care Dressing Procedures", 1997, Cassandra Levescy, LVN III, Alsleben, M.D.. Sponsored by Aloe Life International and chosen for presentation at the 12th Annual Symposium on Wounds Care in Dallas, Texas by Springhouse.

21.) ***BioMarkers-The 10 Keys to Prolonging Vitality, You can control the aging process!,*** 1992, Evans W, P.H.D., Rosenberg IH, M.D.,Professors of Nutrition and Medicine at Tufts University, FIRESIDE.